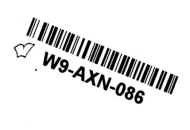
W9-AXN-086

HEALING
ONE CELL AT A TIME

Unlock Your
Genetic Imprint
to Prevent Disease
& Live Healthy

DR. GORDON CROZIER
WITH ANGIE KIESLING

Copyright © 2015 by Dr. Gordon Crozier

Healing One Cell at a Time
by Dr. Gordon Crozier

Printed in the United States of America

ISBN 978-0-692-51226-5

All rights reserved. No part of this document may be reproduced or transmitted in any form, by any means (electronic, photocopying, recording, or otherwise) without the written permission of the author.

Dedication

—⚬—

I want to thank my wonderful wife, Michelle, who has been blessed with wisdom beyond that of study or age. Her constant encouragement to conquer fears and achieve the next goal along with the story of love and courage she has endured continue to inspire me.

Thank you to my family, who has sacrificed while I spent countless hours studying, going to conferences, and devouring webinars and articles. All the time away from them cannot be recouped. It was a sacrifice for all of us.

A special thank you to Ariel and Victoria, my oldest girls, who spent time typing up many rewritten chapters and manuscripts and brought me new, inspiring articles for my continued growth in knowledge.

I love my family and pray we continue to grow in love for one another as we reach out to those who are sick and hurting emotionally, spiritually, and physically so that continual health and healing will be available to many.

Contents

—ᴍ—

Introduction

One Size Does Not Fit All: Genetic-Based Medicine

—〰—

O nce or twice a century, a paradigm shift takes place that turns our world upside down. Right now a seismic shift is shaking the medical field, although many are not aware of it, others ignore its gathering strength, and still others may even oppose it. *Why is this relevant to me*, you may ask. Because the information you're about to read could change your life—maybe even save it.

It's all centered on one underlying truth: your body is so unique, so snowflake-specific, that no other human being is wired exactly like you. And for that reason, medical care for your body should be as tailor-made to *you* as a custom Armani suit. Make no mistake about it: in medicine, as in clothing, one size does not fit all.

Welcome to the emerging field of genetic-based medicine. For years we have tested newborn babies for possible genetic mutations. Over the past years, the fields of DNA profiling and the human genome have exploded with knowledge. Finding specific genes and variants to genes has grown so fast that keeping up with possible treatments in Westernized medicine has not been able to stay abreast of this knowledge.

New discoveries in human genetics have had astounding impact on almost every specialty in medicine and now even on the emerging field of anti-aging medicine. With 76 million Baby Boomers alive today in the United States alone, growing old gracefully has become a serious concern for both men and women—not to mention big business.[1] By 2030 one in five Americans will be older than sixty-five, a reality that will put a strain on our current healthcare system.[2]

But what if I told you that you can not only "grow old gracefully" but also healthfully, with a spring-in-your-step vitality you thought you would never experience again? And what if this radiant health and vitality could be yours not through plastic surgery but by *unlocking your body's own natural healing powers and the fountain of youth imbedded within every cell of your physical makeup.*

Like so many life-changing encounters, I stumbled onto this one almost by accident. It took getting sick for me to be propelled on a journey toward healing and lifelong wellness. And, believe me, when I say "sick" I mean so weak I couldn't crawl off the bed, so ill that everything I ate ran right through my body, so cognitively impaired that for two years I lost the ability to read as a child (you'll read my story in the first two chapters of this book).

The silver lining of my sickly youth is that it led me to find answers in the study of medicine. When I saw that conventional medicine failed to provide the *why* and root-cause cure behind so many diseases; however, my quest for answers led me to what I practice today: integrative, genetic-based medicine. My practice, Excellent Living in Lake Mary, Florida, specializes in treating people who have been sidelined by conventional medicine. Typically, they've tried every therapy, every prescription drug, and every treatment plan known to man—and they're still sick, sometimes to the point of immobility. The good news is that we're seeing recoveries so profound they literally change people's lives.

In the following chapters you will meet several other people who suffered from chronic illnesses, ranging from Lyme disease to parasites to adrenal fatigue, and learn how their physical breakdowns have been transformed into health breakthroughs.

Seeing the Cellular You

If scientists could put you under a microscope, what would they see? Thanks to DNA profiling from simple blood and saliva tests, we're now able to produce multi-page readouts of your entire genetic breakdown—it's you at the cellular level.

This medical technology allows us to see which medicines and macronutrients can be used with a person's specific genetic profile. Although this testing can be rather pricey, it is very beneficial particularly when looking at individual genes and the breakdown of specific medicines.

Genes and DNA have become extremely important in understanding disease and susceptibility to disease. Breakthroughs in these areas and an individual's unique molecular characteristics now hold the promise of customized healthcare and customized anti-aging. In an age of genetically modified foods, produce saturated with pesticides, chemical agents in everything we contact, and EMFs (electromagnetic fields) that alter our bodies' natural biochemical processes, most of us are ticking time bombs, genetically speaking. If the trajectory continues unhindered, our bodies may one day be fertile breeding grounds for disease.

So what is customized individual healthcare or genetic-based medicine? It is using a person's unique molecular characteristics (genetic and epigenetic distinctions) to select treatments customized to that set of molecular variants to optimize the individual's ability for health and to prevent adverse outcomes.

Knowing these variants enables physicians, naturopaths, and other healthcare practitioners to direct a patient into the proper supplements needed, along with avoiding particular supplements and medication that will cause harm or worsening of symptoms.

In my practice, we use all genetic materials, including LabCorp's HLA/DRBQ, to see the individual's ability to process or remove mycotoxins—microfungi that are capable of causing disease and death in humans—from the molecular structures. This is a simple genetic blood test that can reveal intrabody "glitches" with mold, bacteria, and other mycotoxins, fatty acids, low MSH (melanocyte stimulating hormone), and more.

When I combine this along with other genetic testing, I get an entire picture of how an individual may attain health and prevent the effects of possible disease-related symptoms. We cannot "cure" the disease but rather optimize the body so that its own inherent cellular healing takes place.

Never underestimate the body's ability to heal and rejuvenate itself. Among my client base are individuals who could honestly be called walking miracles. But even if your goal is simply to reverse the damaging effects of aging, you've come to the right source, because one inevitable result of cellular healing is protracted youthfulness—sometimes by as much as fifteen or twenty years in appearance.

Whole-body health, youthful vitality, physical and mental wellbeing...these are the essence of what this book is all about. It is my hope that you too will unlock your body's inherent "fountain of youth" and live the life you were meant to live.

Chapter 1

A Stolen Childhood

—◠◠◠—

"Dr. Crozier! Can you hear me?" the nurse shouted, but her voice blended into the background music playing in the operating room.

"Dr. Crozier!" Now I heard it loud and clear, the staccato sound of her voice punching out a rhythm with the beeping heart monitor. My ears rang and I struggled to open my eyes. As the faces of my operating team came into focus, all gazing down at me, I realized with horror what had happened: I had just passed out while performing a gynecological surgery.

I felt the cold tile floor beneath my head and limbs, but something else too—yes, it was *this* that had caused me to pass out. Every joint and muscle of my body screamed in pain. Now I remembered. For the past several months, as I made my rounds, it felt like I was walking on glass. I was foggy-headed and fatigued all the time, but I pushed through for the sake of my patients. Today all the pain had caught up with me, and my body and mind simply checked out.

This was a familiar pain, my old childhood nemesis come to call after years of thinking I had finally escaped its clutches. And of course the reason for its return made sense. Unknown to me at the time, the hospital where I worked in the foothills of eastern Kentucky—a place known for its individualized care and nuns gliding through the corridors—was a toxic breeding ground for black mold.

Mercifully, I had passed out at the very end of the operation, and the intern assisting me was able to close the patient's skin. Two people hoisted me up from the floor and helped me to the break room so I could lie down. As they dimmed the lights and shut the door, one thought ran through my head: *I can't be sick because of what my wife just went through. I have to be healthy for her.* Michelle had lost her first husband to brain cancer; I didn't want to cause her to be a widow for the second time at such a young age.

Desperate for answers, I sought out a friend who knew I was interested in natural healing, although she didn't know how bad off I was. She introduced me to a glutathione accelerator (GSH) supplement, and within three months my symptoms pretty much resolved. That experience changed my whole view—and suddenly I knew what I was going to do with the rest of my life and where I was going to go in medicine.

At fifty-three years of age, I resigned from the medical center in Kentucky to seek training in integrative medicine because now I firmly believed that the body was created to heal itself.

Welcome to My Nightmare

The summer after second grade brought radical changes in my life. As a little boy with white-blond hair, playing in the fields and woods of the flat prairie land, I couldn't foresee that what was about to happen would alter my life forever. But the truth is change had already come. One year earlier my dad, a Baptist church-planting missionary, announced to the family that we were moving yet again—this time to North Dakota. Inwardly I sighed; I knew what that meant: new state, new school, new church, and the challenge of making new friends in a strange new place.

The youngest of four children, I could still remember the sights and sounds of Alaska, where I was born in 1957. And even though I'd had my share of health problems, including the dreaded chicken pox, all I wanted to do was go outside and play. Chasing my friends, I would pedal my bike hard toward the sun as it slid westward in the sky until Mom called me home to supper.

On this particular day, as we rode our bikes for miles and miles around the dirt roads, I'd jumped off at one point to venture into the woods, pretending I was Daniel Boone. I probably didn't even notice that on the ride home I scratched my head a lot. Two days later, when the itch persisted, my mom looked through my hair and found the culprit: a common deer tick, wedged in the very top of my head. Dad lit a match and pulled it out. No harm, no foul. This was par for the course for any kid playing in the woods.

About a week later I came down with flu-like symptoms. My parents were the hardy type, trained to believe you don't really need to go to the doctor—you just suck it up and go on. So I drank a lot of liquids and curled up in my bed, trying to sleep it off. But I was getting worse. When my symptoms finally started to abate, we all figured I had knocked the virus out of my system. However, by the following month the symptoms were not only back, I was much, much worse. Now my skin was turning yellow. After the sclera of my eyes turned yellow too, my parents realized something was seriously wrong with me.

All the medical tests came back negative and the doctor determined I had some type of hepatitis—no doubt caused by a virus of some sort that would eventually wear off. "Keep him away from other children," he told my parents, and sent us home. Slowly over time I felt a little better, but I never felt 100 percent again. I never got back to my baseline.

That fall, when I went back to school, I found I could no longer read. Nothing made sense. I could see words on the page, but they looked like gibberish. Before the strange illness, I had been at the top of my second-grade class, but as I moved into third grade the school's educators placed me in special education—and I failed.

This was horrible for me. I couldn't figure anything out. Taunts of "Hey retard!" echoed down the hall as I walked head down toward the exit door at the end of every school day, blinking back tears. Mrs. Wheeler, my favorite teacher in special education, worked with me tirelessly to help me regain my reading skills. Over time our efforts paid off, but I really could not read functionally again until I was in the sixth grade.

During the next few years I was sick off and on frequently—colds, tonsillitis, flu-like symptoms that kept coming back. I drank a horrible iron liquid to combat anemia, but nothing really worked. I remember getting so excited when my dad announced that the whole family was going to the state fair in Minot that year—finally, something positive on my horizon! But my body had other plans. Instead of heading to the state fair, I landed in the hospital with my tonsils taken out.

Recovering from this surgery, compounded by my vague ongoing illness, I found I just didn't feel like participating as a normal child anymore. In the past I had loved to ride my bike and play outdoors with my friends until twilight, but now I didn't. Everything had changed. I was depressed and didn't realize it, preferring to do something by myself—play with my Lincoln Logs or Matchbox cars, or draw pictures—rather than join in to group activities. The Gordon I had once been was no more.

Little Boy Lost

"Mom!" I grabbed my stomach and rolled over in bed. The sound of my voice had urgency to it, and within minutes my mother flicked on the bedroom light and peered down at me.

"What is it, Gordon?" Her furrowed brow communicated her concern. "It's three o'clock in the morning."

"My stomach hurts bad," I said between wincing breaths. Stabs of pain shot through my abdomen and I cried out again. Fearing the worst—appendicitis—she rustled my dad from bed and they hauled me to the emergency room, but the doctors could find nothing wrong with me. This scene would be repeated several times during my fourth-grade year and beyond, and eventually I was like the boy who cried wolf. Cries of pain in the day or night, or complaints of other bodily aches, met with skepticism, but my parents dutifully took me to the hospital multiple times. My mystery illness confounded every doctor that examined me.

By the sixth grade my abdominal pain was increasing, and now it was accompanied by frequent infections. Various doctors prescribed antibiotics, including high doses of penicillin, and one time the dosage was so high my whole body became stiff and I had shortness of breath—what I now recognize as an extreme allergic reaction. It turns out a lot of this was genetic, but back in the 1960s nobody had ever heard of genetic-based medicine. When I put the pieces together much later as an integrative physician, I realized my young body had the inability to remove mycotoxins.

After that horrible allergic reaction, my depression worsened. I was never a happy child, but suddenly I got much worse. About two weeks after that reaction, I took a rope from my Boy Scout kit and threw it over the curtain rod in my closet, thinking I could hang myself and make everybody's life easier.

My mom walked in as I struggled to tie a noose. "Oh Gordon, stop it!" she said. "Don't be so dramatic. It's not that bad." She thought I was just acting out. Like many kids who suffer alone, I didn't know how to put into words just how wretched my existence had become. I literally wanted to die. Remember, these were the days when you just "pulled yourself up by the bootstraps" and soldiered on. So I went on—still struggling in school, dealing with the chronic pain that wracked my body, and keeping mostly to myself.

As I moved into my teen years, and my family moved to Pennsylvania, a dedicated tutor brought me up to grade level with math and reading, and suddenly I was scholarship material. Miserable in public school, at sixteen I begged my parents to let me attend a prestigious prep school on Long Island where two of my cousins were enrolled. So off I went to boarding school, a place renowned for having the sons of famous fathers on its roster.

Have Money, Will Dabble

A funny thing happens among the boarding-school children of the wealthy. These well-brought-up and very preppy youngsters, usually reared with good moral foundations, suddenly discover a formula previously unknown to them: independence + money = access to drugs.

Even though I was a scholarship student—the "poor relation" among millionaires' sons—I found that rubbing shoulders with the elite crowd opened exciting new vistas to me. For starters, if we had good grades we were allowed to get on the train and ride into New York City for the weekend. We'd go in and romp all over the city in our preppy clothes then come back to campus Sunday night, feeling like men.

One of my classmates, the heir to a huge fortune, introduced me to marijuana and then marijuana laced with PCP. Far from my church roots by now, I couldn't care less about God or anything that had to do with my old life. All I wanted was a place where I could fit in, and maybe, just maybe, I had finally found it.

Because I got really good grades, I was permitted to go on a week-long canoeing trip in the Adirondacks in September 1974, my first year there. My physical strength and symptoms had improved, so I actually had the energy to participate. This seemed like the light at the end of a very long tunnel; finally I felt like I was getting better. But no sooner did we get back than I started having severe abdominal pain—worse than ever before. Profuse bouts of diarrhea followed it.

At home I had always eaten fairly organically. My mom made her own bread, we ate fresh vegetables from a garden, and our water came from a spring. Now, at school, for the first time I ate Fruit Loops, Apple Jacks—all the sugary, processed food that marked the 1970s. Just a few months into the school term, I was losing weight and writhing in pain every night, plagued by insomnia.

Eventually I got so desperate I jumped out of the second-story window of my dorm room onto a flight of cement stairs. Unfortunately I was just bruised. "Are you crazy!" my friend Tommy whispered to me from the dorm window. "This is after-hours. We're gonna get in so much trouble!" He rushed down to the ground floor and helped pick me up off the steps. I didn't realize it then, but I was being kept alive for a purpose. There was a plan for my life (and there's one for your life too!). It's easy to read about a person's life and take it as just a story, but you have to realize I was truly desperate. My health was declining again, and I had no real hope in my life.

The next morning, while singing in a church for the glee club, I had a profound spiritual awakening, and after that I felt such a burden lifted from my shoulders. My pain continued to get worse as time went by, however, so I went to see the school nurse during my junior year. Yet somehow I knew everything was going to be okay. The nurse told my parents I needed to come home because I was losing weight drastically. Whereas before I had been a little chunky, now my weight was down to the low 100s. My parents brought me home at Christmas break, and I knew I wasn't going back to school.

How do you put weight on a kid? You feed him milkshakes! At least that's the "down home" thinking that prevailed in my household. With good intentions, my dad gave me milkshake after milkshake to drink—but they made me sick. My father was just not the type who would easily take you to the doctor. When he was a boy, his parents put him in a wagon and pulled him to school with rheumatic fever. I knew what I was dealing with. Yet the severity of my symptoms won out, and I was in and out of the hospital all that summer after eleventh grade. I would crawl out of bed to paint (I had discovered art as an outlet years before) but that was about it.

Once again, at night the pain was so bad my mom could hear me crying. When I got down to

94 pounds, the doctor put me in the hospital. I had stopped growing a year earlier, at age sixteen. After multiple rigid colonoscopies, the doctors finally got a biopsy that showed I had Crohn's disease, so I was in and out of the hospital (again) for a year. After the diagnosis, they put me on medication, but it didn't do much for me. Back then, nobody knew anything about mold toxicity and that mold is related to bowel dysfunction. So they didn't know what the root of my real problem was.

Plus, remember that tick bite I got when I was eight? Years later I realized I had undiagnosed Lyme disease, compounded by mold toxicity and Crohn's disease—but no one knew the full spectrum of the "dis-ease" that was debilitating my body. The medical team just threw medications at my symptoms, and when they said they wanted to do surgery to remove a large portion of my colon, I thought, *This is ridiculous. I am not going to let them do surgery on me. I'm leaving this place.*

Taking Charge of My Own Health

The day I heard the words "colon surgery" I decided I was going to change my eating. I didn't know this was the cure for what ailed me, but I knew that many foods bothered me. Using a process of deduction, I learned to cut out certain foods, one at a time. For instance, I cut out dairy because every time I ate it I would have explosive diarrhea.

Around the same time, I started doing a lot of juicing with raw vegetables. I ate more raw foods, the way nature made them. I stopped eating all processed foods and cut sugar way back in my diet. If something came from a boxed mix, I wouldn't eat it. If it was natural, it was okay. Every time I would get sick from a particular food, I eliminated it from my diet. At the same time I started taping positive affirmations all over my mirror—and I spoke those affirmations out loud daily, literally speaking health and healing into my life.

By senior year, my body had started to heal itself, but I didn't really notice until after graduation. Bowel movements weren't as bad as before, and I had a bit more energy now. I even started gaining weight. This was a slow process over the course of more than a year, but little by little I was getting better. As part of my newfound regimen, I eliminated all the medications my doctors had prescribed and started taking supplements instead.

After art school and then Bible college I still didn't know what I wanted to do with my life. Several of my relatives were doctors, and I saw people in the Pennsylvania steel mills getting laid off, so I thought *well, people will always be sick*. It made sense.

A New Life Path Opens Up
I made the decision to become a physician's assistant (PA)—someone who would work in the medical field but not have all the stress medical doctors

faced. With my degree in hand, I got a job as a PA in the fields of neurology, neurosurgery, and ophthalmology. Curiously, all the doctors I worked with said the same thing: "Gordon, you're too smart; you need to go back to medical school and become a doctor."

During medical school, my eyes gradually opened to the creativity of combining conventional medicine with integrative medicine. Because of what I had gone through—being chronically ill for most of my growing up years—I knew I wanted to do more than just treat symptoms. I ended up practicing in obstetrics and gynecology for years, including serving as a clinical professor at the University of Kentucky. During my late forties I got involved in the American Academy of Anti-Aging (A4M) and regenerative and functional medicine. Around the same time, roughly 2008, I started seeing the limitations of surgery and conventional medicine. I saw women having hysterectomies for pain unnecessarily. We'd do the surgery and they would still have pain. We sent them for a bowel workup and it wasn't their bowel. Well, what was it?

I had seen the way allopathic medicine was done and how it was just pushing a drug at a symptom; I saw my colleagues doing the same thing. Fighting fatigue, I felt my old symptoms returning, and a physician friend gave me a drug for chronic fatigue syndrome (CFS). I knew the decline in my health was not stress-related because I had had to deal with stress for years. I started looking for alternative measures, something and somebody that integrates natural medicine with our medical culture.

Even as I took two fellowships with A4M, and became board certified, my body started breaking down again. I felt intense burning on the bottoms of my feet and suffered horrible fibromyalgia and CFS symptoms. I had bouts of diarrhea. Everything I experienced as a child was coming back on me. Things got so bad that I actually passed out during a surgery, as recounted in the opening of this chapter.

I know now that I was a victim of extreme mold toxicity—the operating rooms were moldy and I also lived in a moldy house while in Kentucky. This pushed me even more toward the integrative route in medicine. Desperate for answers, I went to a neurosurgeon, a neurologist, a family practitioner, a psychiatrist, an infectious disease specialist, and an internist trying to find out what was wrong with me. It wasn't my diet. I was eating well and had been for years since my childhood illness.

So sick I could barely make it through a day, I was getting ready to go on disability when I had a personal epiphany—a scientific "aha" moment that changed everything. For you see, it was around this time that I realized *my body couldn't remove mycotoxins on its own*. Without that ability, the body goes into a tailspin that may last years or even decades, but eventually all toxicity, unless removed, leads to demise.

Due to the lack of benefit and help from traditional medicine, I began to look into integrative medicine and alternative medicine routes. I found my home and a base for scientific knowledge at A4M—and eventually transitioned completely into this medical practice, leaving obstetrics and gynecology behind.

As I worked alongside influential integrative doctors, I started connecting all the concepts and seeing genetic profiles that explained why people have specific symptoms from certain diseases and why some people will react a certain way and others will not. I realized you could go further than current integrative medicine did, and so I developed a pioneering concept for treatments that is highly individualized according to each person's genetic makeup.

This approach allows me to realize what diet program they should be on, what supplements they can take, and what IV therapies would best suit that specific individual, while all along opening up other methylation pathways in their body to introduce even more healing treatments. (Methylation is the process of replacing a hydrogen ion for a methyl group so that vitamins, minerals, proteins, and amino acids can be utilized in the body correctly.)

Put in simple layman's terms, I now knew how to use certain nutrients in the body so that in places where the light switch had been turned off, suddenly it was turned on and the body could start to heal itself.

Chapter 2

Good Vibrations:
The Key to Healing One Cell
at a Time

—◆—

The Beach Boys Had It Right

Over the past decade, while most of us quietly went about our daily lives, science made some quantum leaps in understanding life at the intra-cellular level. It turns out—remarkably—that cells actually vibrate, and that vibration makes noise. As *Popular Science* once stated, "You have to listen very, very closely, but yes, cells produce a symphony of sounds."[3]

Discoveries such as this get me excited about the future of healthcare, but it's not really surprising to me because I've learned from my relationships with hundreds of patients, not to mention my own healing journey, what a *miraculous organism the human body is*. And not only do cells vibrate, but good cells have a "good" vibration while bad cells have a completely different vibration. And you thought it was just a song from the '60s!

Why do cells have different vibration settings? This has been studied, and we know that good cells have a specific vibration and can therefore take nutrients *into* the cell. Bad cells have a different vibration and actually reject nutrients. A study done[4] showed that certain tones will bring a healing vibration to the body, and, incredibly, we now know that our emotions and self-talk also change the way these cells vibrate.

You Are What You Say (and Think and Feel)

Let me tell you a quick story about one of my patients. This fifty-year-old woman came to me with a diagnosis of multiple sclerosis and Lyme; she even had MRI results showing spirochetes on her brain. At first she improved dramatically on the healing regimen I prescribed for her; even her husband noticed the great improvements. But after a short time she started repeating a particular statement, one of sickness and defeat. The constant verbal statements of "I'm getting worse" stopped her improvements and she began to decline again. She grew bitter when she saw others getting better around her while she was stagnant in her healing process.

Whenever I work with significantly ill individuals, I encourage them to get counseling because many of these people have a PTSD type response. Changing our emotions to be positive ones can in fact *change the very vibration of our cells*. Concentrating on a positive mindset is so important to bringing each cell into a healing mode.

I have found that unforgiveness does not hurt the individuals it is directed at, but instead only hurts the one who is harboring that feeling. Oftentimes the person we have unforgiveness or bitterness toward does not even know of our negative feelings toward them. It doesn't affect them, it affects us. In my own life, when I was holding onto bitterness, it made me tired and unable to maintain an immune response because our immune system is suppressed by these powerful emotions. When I learned to let go of these emotions it opened up the pathways to bring in positive emotions.

Focusing positive emotions and being thankful for what I have—rather than focusing on what I don't have—makes all the difference. Focusing on the negative causes every cell to be focused on death and destruction. I encourage you to make this change in your life. Try it and see what happens. I think you'll be amazed at the transition!

Be gracious with yourself; it will take time to reset your mind. Why? Because it's not about just saying it a couple of times but truly meaning it. As you begin to focus on the positive, it will become your belief system. Your believing will then dictate your living. This is how you can change your cells' vibration to permit healing to begin and continue.

In my practice, Excellent Living, I have developed IV drips that will get these nutrients to the cell. For those unable to travel to obtain these IVs, we plan out a course of oral supplements specific for their genetics and problems, but still addressing the cell function and cell wall. As we "remove and restore," healing begins. This process can be difficult, but it's well worth the journey. As the adrenal gland cells heal, it brings about the normalization of enzymes, and as the gut heals, each cell will then break down and absorb nutrients in the correct form and manner. Likewise, as the cells in our brain heal, they then secrete proper serotonin, dopamine, and other neurotransmitters. Healing genetically from the cell permits whole body healing.

A Peek at the Cellular You

Creating optimal health comes down to the cellular level because if your cells aren't healthy, you aren't healthy. The inverse is also true: healthy cells equal a healthy you, and that's the goal of this book. By the time you turn the last page, I want you to be empowered to take charge of your own health and healing. So let's get started.

Every cell in your body contains many parts:

- Cilia
- Lysosome
- Centriole
- Microtubules
- Golgi apparatus
- Smooth endoplasmic reticulum
- Mitochondrion
- Rough endoplasmic reticulum
- Cytoplasm
- Nucleolus
- Nuclear membrane
- Chromatin
- Ribosome
- Cell membrane

Whether we're talking about the cells in your brain, your gut, your heart, or any other part of your body, these cells are designed to act like micro-computers, telling that body part how to function properly. The problem lies in the fact that toxins get trapped in many areas of the cell, inhibiting normal function. These toxins bombard us from every angle: the processed foods we eat, the environment around us, the lotions and potions we put on our skin and hair, to name a few. Multiply that toxic overload by decades and you can realize why so many people are sick with vague, "untreatable" illnesses.

Each of the fourteen parts to the cell plays a critical role in the cell's function and therefore a function in our bodies. For example, the mitochondria play a big role in our energy and need vitamin B, amino acids, and proper fats to function normally. The mitochondria also form a bilipid layer in the cells, but we in the Western world have eaten the incorrect oils for so long that it has caused the bilipid layer to become fragile. This layer is very susceptible to toxins. When toxins enter this bilipid layer, they cause deformity to the mitochondria, disrupting the process of cellular respiration, which in turn produces ATP (adenosine triphosphate)—the "gasoline" that powers all living things. Over a course of time, this will cause fatigue and/or decreased ability to concentrate or have adequate cognitive power.

Almost the same is true for the cell membrane. The cell membrane is critical because it permits nutrients into the cell and helps waste products be removed from the cell. The bilipid layer of the cell wall is more ridged than the mitochondria; as a result, toxins get stuck in the membrane, causing it to become irregular shaped, thereby altering the sodium potassium channels. When these channels don't function normally, the cells become very sick and can even die. These are the channels on ports permitting nutrients into the cell and removing waste from the cell.

A Toxic Soup
So what kind of toxins can get trapped in these fourteen areas of the cell? Pesticides, herbicides,

incorrect fatty acids, heavy metals; and on top of these may be the toxins introduced by parasites, bacteria, and Lyme. The disruption of these lipid layers can cause severe cell dysfunction, and for that reason restoration must be done very carefully.

I've seen so many doctors, even those using natural methods, give supplements to detox these toxins. But often the toxins will be released from the current areas and then be redistributed to other areas. When they reattach to other areas they become even more difficult to remove. The toxic overload causes the cells to morph, and the activity of the cells is changed. These cells will no longer perform their normal function. For example, a muscle can go into spasm or not function at all, or the serotonin receptors may not function as normal, leading to depression. These are only two small areas that can be affected, but the implications for whole-body breakdown are severe.

Consider what happens when the immune system is debilitated due to cellular toxicity. Toxins can suppress or even *shut down* the immune system, rendering that individual susceptible to every virus or bacteria they come in contact with. Some research has shown that the toxins put off by the Lyme outer coat have suppressed the immune system, or even the flagella from the Lyme (borreliosis) bacteria will cause it to hide from our immune system.

If toxins are removed in an appropriate way, the immune system and almost every cell in our body will begin to function, but for them to function they will also need appropriate fats, amino acids, and minerals to set up the proper healing.

As we'll see in the next chapter, there's also one critical ingredient produced by healthy cells that makes you function like a well-oiled machine. I like to call this substance the Fountain of Youth, because without it our bodies break down—literally age—much faster than nature intended. But it doesn't have to be that way. You can "reverse the curse"!

Chapter 3

Glutathione—the Body's Own Fountain of Youth

—⟨⟨⟨—

For decades scientists have known that glutathione plays a vital role in protecting our cells, tissues, and organs. It's the "stuff" that keeps you youthful, vibrant, and functioning at optimum levels in every part of your body. Found in all plants and animals, glutathione is essential for life, and without it death occurs.

PubMed, the official U.S. government library of medical research, includes nearly 100,000 scientific studies and articles documenting glutathione's benefits to the body. Take a look at the list below and you'll see why this natural antioxidant is so critical to your health and well being.

High glutathione levels give you:

- more energy
- greater stamina
- optimized immune system
- quick recovery from exercise
- razor-sharp mental focus
- sound sleep
- less inflammation
- less joint discomfort
- longevity of life

Glutathione is the master antioxidant known to man, and it also helps all other antioxidants circulate. When scientists have done muscle biopsies on people who aged rapidly, they found low levels of glutathione. Not surprisingly, people who aged more slowly have high levels of glutathione. According to LabCorp, healthy values of around 350 are at the higher end of normal; low levels of glutathione are anything under 150.

Let me give you a vivid picture of how powerful this substance is. I once treated a young model who had gnarled hands from rheumatoid arthritis. After treating her for four months with a powerful glutathione supplement, her hands looked normal again. In her case, rheumatoid arthritis was an inherited trait—her hereditary legacy, so to speak. But I knew she didn't have to accept that debilitating illness as her "new normal." Nor do you have to settle for the aches, pains, and illnesses that may be attacking your life.

What's a Free Radical?

Right now "free radicals" and "antioxidants" are buzzwords in the popular health-and-wellness culture, but what exactly is a free radical, you may be asking. As I mentioned earlier, our bodies are under constant attack from environmental toxins, pollution, stress, and processed foods that wreak havoc by damaging our cells and tissues, interfering with cellular communication and increasing inflammation. Add to that the relentless damage from free radicals, and, over time, your cells can show wear and tear beyond their years.

To cite from one source, "Free radicals are everywhere, in the air, our bodies, and the materials around us. They cause the deterioration of plastics, the fading of paint, the degradation of works of art, aging related illnesses, and can contribute to heart attacks, stroke and cancers. Free radicals are molecules with unpaired electrons. In their quest to find another electron, they are very reactive and cause damage to surrounding molecules."[5]

The Bad News: That "damage to surrounding molecules" is called oxidative stress, and antioxidants are nature's way of detoxifying (or deoxidizing) the damaged cells.

The Good News: Glutathione comes to the rescue. Found and manufactured in every one of our trillions of cells, glutathione can be found in the highest concentrations in our major organs such as the liver, brain, and lungs. It's your body's natural safeguard against accelerated aging.

Although glutathione is created naturally in the body when we're healthy, it easily gets depleted through aging, natural causes, diseases, dehydration, mold, poor diet, pesticides, and stress. When glutathione gets depleted, cellular inflammation increases—setting the stage for disease.

Inflammation is at the root of most diseases, and many illnesses/diseases are associated with low glutathione levels. So as the assault of time, poor diet, stress, and environmental toxins wear us down, we find ourselves without the benefit of this natural cell protector and detoxifier we enjoyed when we were younger.

All of these combined put a heavy toll on our glutathione demand. Ultimately, if there is not enough glutathione in our bodies, our cells, tissues, and organs pay the price.

A Carrier Pigeon for Glutathione

Unfortunately, many of the methods of increasing glutathione are either not effective or insufficient for what our bodies need. A lot of glutathione products come from genetically modified corn, others from fungus (and you already know what I think about that!). Topical, injection, IV, nebulized, oral, liposomal glutathione, or acetyl glutathione—all are poor forms to increase your glutathione levels. The glutathione molecule is very large and hard to get into the cells, and many forms of glutathione supplementation have little effect—maybe a quick fix—while some actually cause glutathione levels to decrease.

The key to increasing glutathione levels is by providing cysteine, a fragile amino acid necessary for our cells to produce glutathione. Simply supplementing cysteine or glutathione orally is ineffective in raising glutathione levels because they are destroyed in the digestion process before they are able to reach the cells.

Enter Riboceine, a breakthrough nutrient compound that acts like a carrier pigeon and takes cysteine into the cell causing the creation of intracellular glutathione to be created. Intracellular GSH is needed, not extracellular like all other forms of GSH. The result of thirty years of study by world-renowned research scientist and medicinal chemist, Herbert T. Nagasawa, PhD, the patented Riboceine molecule combines D-Ribose and cysteine and is released *inside the cell* to create glutathione.

IV glutathione is used in myriad anti-aging centers by a lot of integrative doctors worldwide, but what I found was that these patients' glutathione concentrations were actually *going down* when they were receiving IV treatments. It caused a negative feedback. So when your body has glutathione being pumped in, it shuts down production of more glutathione—the exact opposite of what you want to happen.

I also realized that the glutathione wasn't actually getting into the cells. After time and treating multiple patients, I realized the best form was the Riboceine molecule. So I started to give more of the Riboceine molecule along with IV glutathione (I lowered the dosage and increased the Riboceine taken orally), and when I did this I noticed the patients were getting well.

Healing Ben

One patient named Ben had very high levels of the mold molecule (mycotoxins) in his body. He was not getting better by any of the traditional methods of mold detoxing, but after treatment with IV glutathione and IV lipid resistation, he began to improve dramatically and his levels of the mold molecule went down. There's an FDA standard on what those levels should be, or rather be under, and this patient had fifteen times the normal "allowable" level.

Code	Test	Specimen	Value	Result	Negative if less than	Equivocal if between	Positive if greater or equal
E8501	Ochratoxin A	Urine	6.28 ppb	Positive	1.8 ppb	1.8-2.0 ppb	2.0 ppb
E8502	Aflatoxin Group	Urine	0 ppb	Negative	0.8 ppb	0.8-1.0 ppb	1.0 ppb
E8503	Trichothecene Group	Urine	0.87 ppb	Positive	0.18 ppb	0.18-0.2 ppb	0.2 ppb

Ben also came to me with early Alzheimer's and MS symptoms—and he was only in his thirties. As he started on his treatment program, I watched his cognitive function increase dramatically until he regained 90 percent function. At first he walked with a cane, but gradually he began to walk normally. This treatment plan spanned four months, but whenever I release somebody I always release them with follow-up and supplementation. We often have them come back for future treatments down the road.

A Sticky Paper for Toxins

Toxins like to live in the mitochondria of cells, causing cellular inflammation and all kinds of damage. The result is decreased energy, chronic fatigue, and other chronic maladies. As I already stated, we need intracellular glutathione, not extracellular, because cancers begin with mutations at the cellular level, mostly caused from inflammation (80 percent of cancers have gene mutations due to inflammation). Glutathione acts as a skilled hunter, tracking down those toxins and other cell-killers such as free radicals, removing inflammation in its wake.

Most diseases are associated with inflammation, so you can decrease the activity of that disease by decreasing inflammation at the cellular level. More than ninety diseases are associated with low glutathione levels. Take a look at the mind-boggling list below:

Diseases Associated with Low Glutathione

General
Alcoholism
Endothelial dysfunction
Heavy metal poisoning
Immune signaling
Inflammation

Obesity

Cardiovascular
Angina and spastic angina
Heart attacks
Positive stress tests

Repercussion after cardiac bypass surgery

Unstable angina

Pulmonary

Asthma

Chronic bronchitis

Emphysema (COPD)

Muscle wasting in COPD

Tobacco abuse

Rheumatology

Behcets syndrome

Chronic fatigue syndrome

Fibromyalgia

ME/CFS

Multiple sclerosis

Rheumatoid arthritis

Systemic lupus erythematosis

Systemic sclerosis

Neuro/Psych

ADD

ADHD

Alzheimer's

Anxiety

Autism

Bipolar disease

Depression

Guillain-Barre syndrome

Huntington's chorea

Lou Gehrig's disease (ALS)

Migraine headaches

Multi-infarct dementia

OCD

Parkinson's

Schizophrenia

Dermatology

Acne

Atopic dermatitis

Eczema

Psoriasis

Wrinkles, sagging

Infectious Diseases/ Immunology

Common viral infections (UTI, gastroenteritis)

Hepatitis A, B, and C

Herpes simplex

Herpes zoster/shingles

HIV

Influenza and bird flu

MRSA

Ob/Gyn

Infertility

Spontaneous abortion (miscarriage)

Pre-menstrual syndrome

Oncology

Every cancer studied including:

Brain

Esophagus

Head and neck

Intestine

Kidney

Leukemia (acute and chronic)

Liver

Lung

Lymphoma

Multiple myeloma

Ovarian

Pancreas

Prostate

Stomach

Thyroid

Uterine

Ophthalmology

Cataracts

Macular degeneration

The trouble is, the body is so good at trying to heal itself that the damage from inflammation may go on for *years* before reaching a critical or diseased state—one that's recognizable through traditional diagnosis. Trust me, you don't want to gamble on your health this way. Creating an inflammation-free body is the best way to stave off future disease and illness.

The abbreviated list below will give you an idea of how lethal inflammation is to the human body.[6]

Disease	Mechanism
Allergy	4 Immune Mediated Types + Sensitivities, all of which cause inflammation
Alzheimer's	Chronic inflammation destroys brain cells
Anemia	Inflammatory cytokines attack erythropoietin production

Disease	Mechanism
Ankylosing Spondylitis	Inflammatory cytokines induce autoimmune reactions against joint surfaces
Asthma	Inflammatory cytokines induce autoimmune reactions against airway lining
Autism	Inflammatory cytokines induce autoimmune reactions in the brain arresting right hemisphere development
Arthritis	Inflammatory cytokines destroy joint cartilage and synovial fluid
Carpal Tunnel Syndrome	Chronic inflammation causes excessive muscle tension shortening tendons in the forearm and wrist compressing the nerves.
Celiac	Chronic immune mediated inflammation damages intestinal lining
Crohn's Disease	Chronic immune mediated inflammation damages intestinal lining
Congestive heart failure	Chronic inflammation contributes to heart muscle wasting
Eczema	Chronic inflammation of the gut and liver with poor detoxification and often antibodies against Transglutaminase-3.

Disease	Mechanism
Fibromyalgia	Inflamed connective tissue often food allergy related and exacerbated by secondary nutritional and neurological imbalances.
Fibrosis	Inflammatory cytokines attack traumatized tissue
Gall Bladder Disease	Inflammation of the bile duct or excess cholesterol produced in response to gut inflammation
GERD	Inflammation of the esophagus and digestive tract nearly always food sensitivity and pH driven
Guillain-Barre	Autoimmune attack of the nervous system often triggered by autoimmune response to external stressors such as vaccinations.
Hashimoto's Thyroiditis	Autoimmune reaction originating in the gut triggered by antibodies against thyroid enzymes and proteins
Heart attack	Chronic inflammation contributes to coronary atherosclerosis
Kidney failure	Inflammatory cytokines restrict circulation and damage nephrons and tubules in the kidneys

Disease	Mechanism
Lupus	Inflammatory cytokines induce an autoimmune attack against connective tissue
Multiple Sclerosis	Inflammatory cytokines induce autoimmune reactions against myelin
Neuropathy	Inflammatory cytokines induce autoimmune reactions against myelin and vascular and connective tissues which irritate nerves.
Pancreatitis	Inflammatory cytokines induce pancreatic cell injury
Psoriasis	Chronic inflammation of the gut and liver with poor detoxification
Polymyalgia Rheumatica	Inflammatory cytokines induce autoimmune reactions against muscles and connective tissue
Rheumatoid Arthritis	Inflammatory cytokines induce autoimmune reactions against joints
Scleroderma	Inflammatory cytokines induce an autoimmune attack against connective tissue
Stroke	Chronic inflammation promoted thromboembolic events
Surgical complications	Inflammatory cytokines (often pre-dating the surgery) slow or prevent healing

Unblocking the Pathways

I learned about glutathione in the late 2000s and began to study the importance of it. That's why I now include it in every treatment plan I customize for my patients. Some of the highest concentrations of glutathione are in our liver because the liver is our major detoxification organ—everything is broken down either there or through the kidneys.

A lot of anti-aging centers will say you need to do a liver cleanse and then provide supplements to clean the liver, but in fact the patient is just getting supplements that do very little to cleanse the liver. Glutathione will pull out heavy metals, pesticides—any pollutants we put in our bodies, it's going to attach to it and pull it out through urine or feces or sweat or respiration. It almost acts like a sticky paper that other molecules will attach to and be pulled out of the cells.

If you don't have your glutathione levels corrected, you won't even begin to have proper methylation, a process by which a hydrogen ion is removed from the cell and replaced with a methyl group. You need a methyl group to utilize certain vitamins, for detoxification, and for all the biochemical pathways to operate correctly.

I can't overstate this: the key to why so many people are so sick is glutathione. Toxins cause genetic glitches and block up the pathways. Glutathione unblocks those pathways.

In the chapters that follow, we'll take a look at the predominant diseases of the twenty-first century that may be claiming the health of you or someone you know—and how to win your health back one cell at a time.

Chapter 4

Unraveling the Gut/ Brain Relationship

—ɯᴜ—

The ancient Greek physician Hippocrates is credited with the well-known phrase "health begins in the colon." Nobody struggles with this, but few people realize there's a connection between the health of your *gut* (intestines) and the health of your *brain*.

Traditional physicians are not recognizing the gut/brain relationship whereas alternative and integrative doctors are constantly looking into the deeper issues of *dis*ease. Years ago a medical journal published an article theorizing that serotonin actually starts in the gut. This translates into help for individual depression—but the implications go much further than that. Even the International Foundation for Gastrointestinal Disorders is noting the relationship between psychological symptoms and IBS. Newer articles concur with this. One of many is the April 9, 2015, issue of the journal *Cell* which showed that 90 percent of serotonin is made in the digestive tract.[7]

With the amount of processed foods we consume and the toxic environments we live in, it's no wonder that serious gut ailments are on the rise. And, sadly, we're seeing younger and younger patients affected by these health and vitality stealers.

A Walking Skeleton
Billy's physical appearance shocked me when he first came in for treatment—at six-feet-one, he weighed only ninety-seven pounds. He had already been to several doctors and was taking Humira, the latest in a string of medications prescribed for Crohn's disease. One drug made him so lethargic he didn't feel like getting out of bed. Just eighteen years old, he was declining fast when a friend suggested he schedule a consultation with me.

Billy told me he had no energy and suffered significant abdominal pain, with about ten watery bowel movements a day. As part of his treatment, we began with a full genetic profile so I could tailor his treatment plan accordingly. Right away I could see that he had a high level of immunoglobulin A (IgA)—an antibody found in high concentrations in the mucous membranes, particularly those lining the respiratory passages and gastrointestinal tract—in his blood. He also tested positive for mycotoxins and for the gene HLA-DRBQ, or the inability to *remove* mold and mycotoxins. Armed with this information, I had a clear picture of why Billy was so sick, and why the drugs only made him sicker.

As we started Billy on treatment, he received very few IV treatments due to being so sick and unable to travel from Nashville all the time. He came several times and we worked with oral supplements instead. After slow gains at first, he began to take off and regain muscle mass. Currently, Billy has been able to start college and has gained forty-five pounds. He reports minimal abdominal pain and has only three bowel movements a day. His words to me: "I now have my life back."

Guts Gone Awry

Your gut is made of an incredibly large and intricate semi-permeable lining. It's also incredibly resilient, but when the intestinal lining is repeatedly damaged due to poor diet, mycotoxins, high levels of the stress hormone cortisol, and other factors, it responds with inflammation, allergic reactions, and other symptoms associated with disease.

One such disease, called **Crohn's disease**, is a painful inflammatory bowel disease that affects between 400,000 and 600,000 individuals in North America. This disease is a multi-factorial ailment caused by bacterial, environmental, immunological, and genetic factors—as you can imagine, not an easy fix. The body's autoimmune system will attack the intestinal tract anywhere from the mouth to the anus. Although there are no known causes, there are a variety of treatment options.

Another increasingly common ailment is **IBS or irritable bowel syndrome,** sometimes called spastic colon. Like Crohn's, it is associated with abdominal pain and diarrhea alternating with constipation, bloating, and flatulence. There is no known cause or single cause. IBS is often more likely to occur after an infection or even after an extremely stressful event. Usually an IBS diagnosis is given on the basis of symptoms alone. This is primarily due to the fact that routine testing seems to produce no abnormalities. The treatments available have had little effect on the patients I see, but there are different treatments available.

The first treatment is usually dietary changes. It appears that different diets work best for different individuals. Some, although lacking in true celiac disease, benefit from a dairy-free diet, but this is not for everyone. According to some articles on PubMed there is a correlation between mold and Crohn's as well as bowel problems. Trichothecene (a fungi mycotoxin) has been noted to cause severe gastrointestinal problems and, when used in chemical warfare, is associated with vomiting and severe bowel bleeding, even causing death.

From GI Distress to Mental Distress

Depression disorders are illnesses of the brain. MRIs have shown that the brain of a depressed person looks different from the brain of a non-depressed individual. The causes may be numerous, but medical science can now prove that *some depression may be related to bowel or GI issues*. Common signs or symptoms of depression are below:

- Persistent sadness, anxiousness, or empty feelings
- Feelings of hopelessness, pessimism
- Feelings of guilt, helplessness, worthlessness
- Irritability, restlessness
- Loss of interest in activities or hobbies (including sex)
- Fatigue and decreased energy
- Difficulty concentrating, remembering details
- Insomnia or excessive sleeping
- Overeating, sometimes loss of appetite
- Thoughts of suicide
- Aches, pains, headaches, cramps
- Digestive problems

Although not every depressed person has bowel-related problems, there is a crossover between many illnesses and depression. This possibly could be related to genetics or inappropriate precursors or enzymes needed for neurotransmitters (Dr. Amen is a great expert on neurotransmitters). And while anxiety may be associated with some bowel or IBS patients, not all anxiety is related to bowel syndromes. Likewise, not all of those who experience anxiety also suffer from depression—but many do.

When emotional distress does accompany IBS or Crohn's, it may cause a worsening of the IBS/Crohn's symptoms. Also, it is not uncommon for people with IBS to develop worsening symptoms while eating at restaurants and social gatherings. Those symptoms may include anxiety due to the *anticipation* that there could be a problem. This unwanted anxiety in turn could develop worsening of symptoms. Now we have a vicious cycle that sets up the IBS and then the anxiety worsening the IBS.

Stressful events are known to affect bowel habits or changes in bowel function. Examples are death, loss of a job, unwanted stress, or even arguments. These can all cause diarrhea and/or constipation and abdominal pain, even in individuals without known IBS. I believe these issues must be addressed in a manner that helps the psychological as well as the physical.

Depression and anxiety can exist without bowel disease such as Crohn's, ulcerative colitis, or IBS. On occasion we may all feel blue or sad, but these feelings are usually short lived and in normal conditions pass in two to four days. For children these feelings usually pass much quicker, and it is very unusual for a child to attempt suicide such as in my story. Back in my day, depression was just something to cope with; in a time renowned for the "perfect family," depression was definitely not something individuals sought help for.

There are several forms of depression disorders:

- Major depression
- Persistent depressive disorder
- Psychotic depression
- Post-partum depression
- Seasonal affective disorder

If you suffer from depression, it may be a good idea to rule out the gut/brain relationship first (with the help of a good integrative physician) before taking an antidepressant. Consider the following story.

Zombie No More

At age twenty-eight, Jamie had suffered from depression for almost ten years. Her history of prescribed drugs read like a pharmacy shelf: Zoloft, Prozac, Abilify, and other antidepressants along with SSRIs. After taking the medications, however, she gradually became aware that she felt like a zombie—numbed out and almost devoid of emotion.

"My friends would tease me and call me zombified," says Jamie, "and when I was in this mental state I cared little about good or bad. I had so little emotion that I could even experience death and not react much. A good friend died in a horrible car accident, and I wish I could have felt the hurt I needed to, but I couldn't feel anything. I was zombified."

Yearning for a "different way of life," she heard me speaking one day, and after the lecture she approached me and shared her story. I listened.

When Jamie first started treatments at Excellent Living, she assured me she didn't have any bowel problems, but in fact I was able to identify that her depression was linked to her bowel functions. After doing a stool test, I realized that she had something called "small intestinal bacterial overgrowth"—an accumulation of incorrect bacteria in the small intestine. Since this is where serotonin production begins, we corrected this and Jamie gradually reported feelings that were normal.

Her customized treatment plan included specific herbal supplements for her bowels. Once that was corrected, I gave her a product that contains 5HTP in very small amounts (for her brain function) because she was on Zoloft, and we had to watch this to avoid "serotonin crisis." After completing some IV therapies with amino acids and fats, Jamie told me she stopped taking Zoloft because it did nothing for her and she felt better without it. Mission accomplished!

Take Your Life Back

Anxiety affects about forty million Americans over the age of eighteen. Panic disorders are related to anxiety, but on the extreme side. Panic attacks can occur at any time, even during sleep. It is estimated that about six million adults are affected by panic disorders. Some with consistent recurrent panic disorders have become completely disabled, unable to perform even normal tasks.

I have seen depression, anxiety, and panic disorders reversed with optimization. On the flipside, I have seen individuals who were almost completely optimized suddenly go to physicians in California or Colorado and be prescribed medical marijuana, only to have everything we accomplished be completely undone.

One of my patients decided to fly out to see a celebrated physician, who prescribed him medical marijuana. This patient became so psychotic he was admitted to a psych ward for about one week. Let me state clearly that I am not against marijuana for medical reasons, but it must be used in a responsible way.

These patients, as well as others I have seen who have bad reactions, usually have a genetic glitch in what we call the "gads." These are a group of epigenetic mutations that has been shown to affect anxiety in some individuals. As I pore over my patients' genetic profiles, I look for patterns—and

I have seen many suffering from anxiety who all share the same genetic profile.

Fortunately, I have been able to optimize these individuals first with IV treatments followed by supplements and fat revitalization; I request that they get counseling along with this treatment.

IDENTITY RECLAIMED

I don't want my identity to be known because I have seen so many chronically ill people lose their jobs and be unable to work. I have told my employees that it was my need to care for my wife that made me get better, but in fact it was the other way around. I did some of my work remotely, but due to severe cognitive problems secondary to Lyme disease I was unable to work.

One day I was driving to the store when I suddenly couldn't recall where I was going and what I was doing. I pulled my car over somewhere in the Philadelphia area and sat there for a while, staring into space. Someone came up, tapped on the window, and asked if I was okay, but I really didn't know if I was or not. He took my phone and called my father. My father and my wife came to get me, and I couldn't believe I didn't know where I was.

Prior to this day I had always been active. I ran, hiked, biked, and even did some mountain climbing. We always went snow skiing in the winter and water skiing in the summer. Since we had some relatives

---

who worked at a famous hospital, my wife took me there. I had a battery of tests during my one week there. The final diagnosis was "relapsing amnesia of unknown cause." They suggested that I start paperwork for disability.

Over the next week I went back to work but began having severe joint pain as well as burning along my spine and legs. This burning was so intense at times that I could not stand anything to touch my skin. Cognitively, I was able to function, but very slowly. As time went on, my health continued to decline.

Unable to help me, my family doctor referred me to a psychologist; he could not help either. My wife found a doctor in New York City that saw me and eventually gave me the diagnosis of Lyme disease. What Lyme disease? I didn't remember a tick bite; I didn't remember having a rash—nothing! This did not make sense to me.

Regardless, I started the intense oral and IV antibiotics he recommended, but this regimen did not work well for me at all. At first I seemed to get better; however, after about one week I started going downhill fast. I developed fasciculation in my legs and the pain increased. By now I was on ten-plus medications and my health was in a tailspin.

I had relatives who knew of Dr. Crozier so we gave him a call. He did a lot of testing, and we found out by an IGeneX test that I did have Lyme as well as the Bartonella bacteria. He discussed how sometimes antibodies, although needed, can combine with spirochete cell membranes to produce incredibly potent toxins, and this was why I had become worse.

My inflammatory levels were really high and all my labs were abnormal.

Upon arriving to see Dr. Crozier, I had just finished six months of IV and oral antibiotics. This regimen had destroyed the beneficial gut flora I was supposed to have in my GI tract. I continued to decline until my second week into Dr. Crozier's treatment, which included colonics with probiotics to help my GI disturbances. Going very slowly, he started me on a limited number of supplements and IV treatments. Little by little, he increased the volume and pacing of treatments—and I gradually got better.

After eight weeks of treatment, I was almost completely back to normal. As of this writing I have been back only one time for a three-day course, which greatly helped me. I am working full time again now and have been advanced to CEO of a large competitive company. I feel I owe my life to Dr. Crozier. My wonderful wife, who was my care-giver, helped me through those several years of what I call total hell. Thanks to those two, I got my life back.

It never ceases to amaze me how optimizing the genetics and healing the cells allows chronically ill patients to take their lives back. Watching their transformation from sickly, wasted individuals to vibrant, healthy participants in life is incredibly rewarding.

Chapter 5

The Unknown Plague: The Ugly Truth about Black Mold

—⚏—

Sherri was a fifty-year-old woman, wife, and mother who worked part-time as a cosmetologist. At the time she came to me she had a significant fatigue rating: ten out of ten (based on exclusion questions/symptoms). She also had significant interstitial cystitis and was seeing a urologist every two or three months, taking pain meds and having routine bladder work done with medication inserted directly into her bladder.

She told me she felt like she couldn't go on anymore. The pain from her IC had become so debilitating that she stopped her part-time job; fortunately, she had a housekeeper and nanny to help with all the household chores.

Sherri wept as I examined her because the pain in her bladder was so intense she could not even permit me to do a complete exam. As I went over her labs, I realized she had the HLA-DRBQ gene, indicating her body had the inability to remove mycotoxins on its own. She also had a defect for fatty acids. Her C-reactive protein levels were so high I could barely understand how someone else would miss this critical lab value. The bottom line: Sherri was suffering the debilitating effects of extreme mold toxicity.

I began to optimize her, taking into account her CBS genetic pathways, and optimized each cell. Sherri gradually improved and stopped all pain medication on her own. This treatment plan was done slowly, and now she only sees the urologist twice a year.

A Hiding Culprit

I call black mold poisoning the unknown plague. Why is sickness on the rise in the United States and throughout the industrialized world? I believe the common theme is biotoxins, a generic term for any toxin originating from a living organism—plant, animal, fungi, bacteria, etc.

Compounding the problem is the chemical load that saturates our environment. From 1930-2000, the global production of chemicals increased from 1 million to 400 million tons each year. These toxic chemicals find their way into our drinking water, our food supply, the products we put on our skin and hair, and the very air we breathe. So we are bombarded with chemicals *and* biotoxins.

Black mold is one of the deadliest biotoxins on the planet and is associated with thirty-six diseases, including Parkinson's, ALS (Lou Gehrig's disease), multiple sclerosis, hormonal deficiencies, colitis, and chronic fatigue syndrome. These illnesses can arise from mold toxicity or just plain mold exposure.

Mold-Associated Diseases

ADD/ADHD
Allergies
Alzheimer's
Anxiety
Blindness
Breathing disorders
Cancer
Chronic bronchitis
Chronic coughing
Chronic sinitus
Crohn's disease
Cognitive decline
Constant headaches
Constipation
Death
Depression
Diarrhea
Ear infections and pain
Epilepsy

Fatigue
Fibromyalgia
Hair loss
Hypersensitivity
IBS
Joint pain
Loss of appetite
Macular degeneration
Memory loss (short- and long-term)
Muscle pain
Nausea
Nose bleeds
Open sores
Parkinson's
Sexual dysfunction
Skin rashes
Vomiting
Weight loss

Mold and mycotoxins are so strong they actually cause an individual's epigenetics to change, and they are very difficult to remove from our bodies. These toxins will also cause us to express genes for certain diseases that may not have been expressing in the past. Think of this process as a flip-switch suddenly being turned on.

For example, let's say your epigenetics show a tendency for colon cancer to develop. As long as that gene is suppressed or not activated, you remain healthy, but if that gene is "turned on" by toxins, it can trigger your body to develop colon cancer, first by hampering your immune system, and then by allowing the cancer cells to metabolize and flourish. Those toxins make you highly susceptible to infections and other diseases as well.

Through my years as an integrative physician, I've seen that most people who suffer with chronic diseases or illnesses have a genetic glitch with their HLA-DRBQ gene. If this gene is absent or mutated, it can prevent the body's natural removal of all mycotoxins.

In November 2002, ABC's *20/20* news television program investigated "the fear and the facts about toxic mold," bringing to light a subject that had been ignored for decades. Suddenly, millions of TV viewers knew this was a topic to be taken seriously. Most notably, the program revealed how black mold exposure can cause respiratory problems such as asthma.

Many people don't realize that mold can even be found in some of our foods, such as coffee. I love my coffee, so I buy coffee that's grown in higher elevations to reduce the likelihood of mold infestation. I also live in Florida—a state known for its high humidity and resulting proliferation of black mold and mildew.

Sick Buildings, Sick Bodies

It's no secret that mold can be found in our homes and buildings. Perhaps you've heard the term "sick building." This modern phenomenon can wreak havoc on our bodies. We work in heated and air conditioned buildings; we live in heated and air conditioned buildings. No longer do we have open circulation with the diluted toxins from outside, but we now recycle all the toxins in these buildings. Air conditioning also brings condensation, increasing moisture, which fungi (mold) love.) In contrast, when we go outside, chemicals and mycotoxins are diluted in the air.

A little water leak that we don't even know about can grow into black mold, turning our bathroom or kitchen or roofline into a breeding ground for a biotoxin that literally poisons us over time. The only thing that gets rid of mold poisoning in the body is glutathione—the cell's own powerful antioxidant—but, paradoxically, mold toxicity depletes glutathione.

Water intrusion can occur even before your house is finished through plywood left out to get wet, for example. Today, with quick construction, many expensive roofs leak in valleys or around flashing. Poor construction can result in water leakage secondary to poor sealing. Flooding basements can cause mold issues, and even just damp dark basements and other areas with water intrusion permit mold to grow. The mold will continue to grow and produce spores, which combine with other toxins from our homes and workplaces. These then become deadly to our bodies.

How do these molds grow? They grow on paper, insulation, wood, primer, plywood, and carpet. Warmth and humidity create a perfect environment for mold to grow and produce spores and gases. We in turn breathe in the gases, making us sick.

Years ago my family and I were excited to move into a new home. Turning the key ushered us into a beautiful space with that fresh-paint smell and thick, plush carpeting. Eager to set up residence, we went about the business of turning our house into a home. But after a few weeks something odd happened. I had pains in my legs and feet that became so intense I had to see many doctors. We knew there was something wrong with the house and found out it was full of mold.

Sadly enough, I see a lot of teachers who are sick. When treated and examined, the main cause is mold. Many schools are infested with mold, which causes our taxes to go up due to disability for teachers. On top of that, our children are exposed to these mycotoxins. The children we see in our practice often have a host of "inexplicable" symptoms including ADD/ADHD and other neurological disorders.

The incidence of learning disorders such as ADD/ADHD has been increasing in recent years. Is this due to schools with flat roofs and decreasing funds available to fix the sick buildings? These gases inside buildings will not only bring down our children, but may also cause many in the corporate world to become disabled and have decreased ability to concentrate and work efficiently.

PubMed includes more than eighty-nine articles on the neurological effects of mold. Research has shown that there is a direct correlation between mold and ALS, Alzheimer's, brain tumors (i.e. glioblastomas), degenerating neurological disorders, multiple sclerosis), Parkinson's, and many other diseases.

I have treated teenagers and adults with tremors, many of whom came to me with no diagnosis. Some were diagnosed with Parkinson's, but many others have had MRIs, CT scans, and PET scans all showing nothing wrong; some showed areas of demyelination not correlating with MS. Not one of these individuals had any testing for mold toxicity.

In my practice, I use the Hooper Lab (Department of Immunology) at the University of Texas Southwestern Medical Center in Dallas to test for an individual's mold levels. A few of these patients may have had a false negative mold test because the mold is trapped. Yes, mold can actually be trapped in the lipid layers of all cell membranes as well as in your bones. Those with neurological diseases can in fact have a significant toxin load in their myelin sheaths, causing destruction of the myelin. When the myelin is destroyed, the conduction of nerve impulses is slowed. This may cause a sense of numbness, tingling, or many other conditions.

Mycotoxins in the brain can cause slowing of the thought process. Demyelination of the peripheral nerves, the nerves not in the brain, can cause the inability to control or move a particular area of the body, such as an arm or leg.

Once again, I turn to PubMed to see what is being recorded in the annals of medical science: over 100,000 articles on mold and brain tumors, 52 articles on mold and glioblastoma (of which only eight are applicable), and 41 showing how the gas from mycotoxins amplifies genes in the nervous system tumors. This means that the gases from mold will cause the genes from any neurological tumor to be amplified and cause them to grow. Mold toxins cause all these things to grow more rapidly.

Many people may have a tumor live and die without even knowing they have it, but if someone is exposed to mold toxins and cannot clear them from their body, they will be the ones who develop tumors that grow, causing a rapid decline. Being exposed to more chemicals, electronic impulses, and mold toxins will push our bodies in a downward spiral, causing one or more of these neurological diseases.

From the Head Down

Why do I take on this subject? I believe everything starts with your genetics. Your genetics influence your brain and the brain controls every part of the body. I believe that everything starts from the head down. The brain controls every part of our body, both sympathetic and parasympathetic systems. The pituitary gland, a very small part of our brain, controls our hormones. The brain controls our heart (cardiac) function, depression, anxiety, insomnia, and so forth. (Wikipedia defines the sympathetic and parasympathetic nervous systems as the two main parts of the autonomic nervous system. They regulate the unconscious actions. The sympathetic nervous system stimulates the body's fight-or-flight response. They are complementary to one another and must work in harmony.)

All of our emotional states begin with the brain. The brain is needed for a positive feeling, and without that positive feeling we will never be well. This is in fact part of our healing. However, genetics trump this and will actually heal or cause our neurological condition to decline.

Neurological conditions are also important to me because people in my life have been affected. Personally, I fought depression, tremors, and syncope most of my childhood years. My father, aunts, and uncles all were diagnosed with Alzheimer's and dementia. Seeing peoples' lives ripped from them in so many different ways affected me profoundly. My wife's late husband died at the age of thirty-three from a brain tumor (glioblastoma), leaving her and their four children to struggle with the why. After healing and repairing, my wife has come alongside me to help in bringing a voice of health to everyone we can touch.

Diseases associated with mold exposure include: allergies, abnormalities of the autoimmune and autonomic systems, asthma, autism, emphysema, Alzheimer's, anxiety, anemia, possible CLL, dementia, depression, demyelization, eye problems from demyelization, cataracts and retinal detachments, eczema, fatigue, fibromyalgia, headaches, migraines, MS, Parkinson's, GI disturbances, Crohn's, ulcerative colitis, IBS, hormonal imbalance, premature menopause, infertility, early andropause, thyroid or hypothyroid problems, growth hormone, and many other problems. I am not saying that mold is the only cause of these diseases/illnesses, but there is a very high probability that it was involved.

Why Don't We Take Mold Seriously?

If mold can be an issue with so many diseases, then why don't we take it more seriously? I personally have had effects from one or more of these issues in the past and probably could have qualified for disability because of them. Being a determined person, and having grown up in a family with high work ethics, I did not choose that route but instead chose to find the cause and eliminate the mold toxins from my life—or at least learn how to optimize my body. I learned how to work with my genetics and my inability to remove mycotoxins (on my own) for cellular health and healing.

I've treated people who were on supplemental hormones, but when the mycotoxins were removed the need for hormones stopped. One young man, college aged, was so sick he was unable to eat food and was being kept alive by a PICC line. He didn't realize he had an issue with mold, but after a short period of time of being optimized through treatment, he was able to start eating, his body absorbed food naturally, and he continued to improve and gain weight.

Some people, including myself, have noticed that being around mold will make them nauseated. This is the black mold causing irritation of the gastrointestinal lining. When this lining becomes irritated and inflamed, it stops absorbing the nutrients the individual needs for basic health and begins to absorb the things that need to be excreted—things like gluten (the inflammatory parts of wheat), which causes abnormal gliadin antibodies to form.

Over time, so many people with irritated GI linings will develop allergies to many foods. The foods eaten most frequently, and those with higher inflammatory markers, are the ones that will cause the most problems.

Mold affecting the GI tract, known or unknown, can cause increased inflammation throughout the body, triggering everything from increased arthritis (joint inflammation) to increased build-up of plaque in the arteries. Mycotoxins have had such a vast effect on everyone and every part of our bodies that I believe we need to focus on this deadly myco-toxin more than we have to date.

Rooting Out the Monster

Can mold be detected in humans? Dr. Hooper of Hooper Lab and RealTime Labs has done an amazing job of studying and identifying mold in the body. Dr. Hooper performed a study revealing that one could test for mycotoxins in the body, including tricoth-esene, aflatoxins, and ochratoxins (this article is available on PubMed). In my own practice, I use RealTime Labs to test for mycotoxins via the urine. If the mycotoxins are trapped in the cell membranes, muscle tissue, bones, or biofilm, the test may have a false low value. I always retest when I am detoxing someone and have seen some values go extremely high—proving that they have mycotoxicity after all.

I also use genetic testing to see who is more likely to be affected by this threat, and it will be those with the HLA genetic, defined as someone who cannot remove mycotoxins from their bodies. LabCorp does a good job of this genetic testing as well, and there are other studies that can show neurotoxicity, bile, cardiovascular, and GI toxicity.

Wait … There's Mold in Our Food?

Mold and mycotoxins are also found in the very foods we eat. A lot of individuals may know about grains and coffees, but I am going to talk about citric acid. Citric acid is developed as a food preservative by a very deadly mechanism for some of us. Citric acid today is not derived from lemons, limes, and other citrus fruits as you would think, but comes from black mold. Why? Because black mold is cheap and will convert sugars to citric acid!

In the manufacturing process, these black molds are fed glucose and sucrose derived from corn starches. We have two bad things going on here: 1) these corns are genetically modified (GMO) and 2) the citric acid is derived from black mold. Citric acid is considered to be harmless as an additive by all food-regulating agencies, but what if there are mycotoxins in these products? What about individuals with gastric reflux or those with allergic reactions?

You may ask when and why all this changed. Well, prior to World War I the food industry used citric acid from citrus fruit. That changed after they found it cheaper to produce citric acid from black mold. What products have this compound in it? Below are just a few examples of products that have citric acid derived from black mold:

- Ketchup
- Cake mixes
- Caramel
- Certain cheeses
- Ice cream, sorbet, and frozen yogurts
- Many canned foods
- Frozen fish (i.e. herring, shrimp, and crab)
- Processed sweets
- Precut packaged fruits and vegetables
- Baby food

What about our supplements? Some supplements will have citrus acid in them, but worse are the digestive enzymes with this compound. Some enzymes are added to foods, including supplements, to aid in our digestion. These digestive enzymes are derived from aspergillus mold. Many digestive enzymes that are recommended daily by integrative doctors could in fact be derived from mold. Thankfully, some companies have realized the potential problem and taken extra steps to filter out all fungal matter from their supplements.

Just remember not all supplements are created equal.

Fighting Your Way Back
What do you do if you think you are sick from mycotoxins or mold? Some people have used cholestyramine or charcoal, but these are only effective in the GI tract. All these toxins get trapped in our

body. About 98 percent of our corn is genetically modified, and so the body recognizes it as gluten molecules, which are very difficult to metabolize.

The bilipid layer of cells is where toxins get trapped, and they distort the channels with the positive/negative ions that take nutrients into the cells so they can divide and absorb like normal healthy cells should do. Adrenals, brain, kidney, heart—every cell in our body needs to live and be healthy.

By now I may sound like a glitchy audio loop, but I believe *increasing intracellular glutathione* to detox these dangerous toxins is the only way one can truly be helped. Glutathione is one of the best heavy metal detoxifiers, so we need our levels up, and the only way we're going to get adequate gluta-thione levels is through that Riboceine molecule we discussed in chapter 3.

So many people are talking about methylation and methylation pathways today, but if those path-ways are not functioning properly then the cells can't absorb the nutrients.

As always, I like to point you toward a healing path every chance I get.

MUGGED BY MOLD

My name is Bruce. Now in my mid-forties, I have been a hard worker all my life. I develop companies and then turn around and sell them. Because this has been a large part of my life, I traveled all around the world.

I had been experiencing some slipping of my thoughts—forgetting words, forgetting times, and sometimes waking up wondering where I was. I also had increased joint pains throughout all the major joints and could hardly stand to workout anymore. Add to that a thirty-pound weight gain and I was pretty much beginning to feel much older than my age.

When I saw Dr. Crozier, I thought I would have a Lyme diagnosis. In fact, I had been told I probably did have Lyme and went to another physician previously but was told no, I didn't have Lyme. She said what I had was probably more psychological in nature, and she referred me to a psychologist instead.

The psychologist did a full evaluation and found nothing wrong with me. He said I was not depressed. He then referred me back to my family doctor, who started me on medication for my fatigue but gave me nothing for the joint pain. The medication made my heart flutter, and I also developed high blood pressure.

The entire time this was going on I continued to decline, getting generalized pain and then more joint pain. I now had fatigue I could not even describe, forcing me to take time off work due to forgetting too much. I really couldn't believe how bad this was becoming.

A relative told me about Dr. Crozier, and I called his office the next day. We did close to thirty-two vials of blood; the lab thought I was crazy and I thought Dr. Crozier was a little nuts for having me get this much blood work done.

He accumulated all the results and said, "I know exactly what your problem is." I flew out to see him, and we spent one and a half hours going over all the results. He showed me how I had the HLA-DRBQ gene, which means an inability to remove mycotoxins—or the gases put off by mold.

I am so thankful for Dr. Crozier; he saved my life and gave me my life back. I now have no blood pressure issues, I have energy, and my pain is dramatically reduced. The treatment program he had me on helped me immensely. He also showed me how to continue the rest of my life with optimizing my cells and helping my body to heal.

Chapter 6

Pervasive Pain: Kicking Fibromyalgia to the Curb

—ɯɯ—

Decades ago, most people had never even heard the word *fibromyalgia,* that strange disorder categorized by chronic widespread pain as well as heightened and painful response to pressure. But now it has almost become a buzzword, so widespread is this illness—especially among women.

Other symptoms associated with this syndrome, which is typically a diagnosis of exclusion, include debilitating fatigue, sleep disturbance, joint stiffness, and difficulty swallowing. Some individuals have noted anxiety, stress-related disorders much like TSD (traumatic stress disorder), numbness, and tingling as well as cognitive disorders. As if those weren't bad enough, fibromyalgia also frequently has psychiatric conditions. Altogether, this mystery malaise can become quite difficult to manage.

Patients may not have all symptoms; they may only have a few. One particular symptom seen frequently that crosses over into many other disorders including mold exposure is short- and long-term memory loss. Some symptoms attributed to fibromyalgia may actually be due to comorbid disorders such as myofascial pain syndrome, diffuse non-detrimental paresthesia, IBS, as well as other gastrointestinal and genital urinary symptoms, including vulvodynia.

Differences in psychological and autonomic nervous system profiles in affected patients can indicate four types of fibromyalgia:

- Extreme sensitivity to pain with no associated psychiatric conditions
- Fibromyalgia and comorbid, pain-related depression
- Depression with concomitant fibromyalgia syndrome
- Fibromyalgia due to somatization

Fibromyalgia has been recognized as a diagnosable disorder by the U.S. National Institutes of Health and the American College of Rheumatology. Despite being a recognized diagnosis, controversy remains as to the cause and nature of fibromyalgia. In my experience, fibromyalgia sufferers are often viewed with skepticism by those in the medical field as well as non-medical fields. I've lost count of the number of times a patient has come to me as a last resort, saying, "Every doctor I've seen thinks this is all in my head. I'm ready to give up hope!"

Women in the Bull's-Eye

Although fibromyalgia affects about 80 percent of the population, it disproportionately attacks women—at a ratio of 7:1 (seven women to every one man). However, recently men's numbers have been increasing, most likely due to environmental factors, which we'll look at shortly.

Dr. Frederick Wolfe, a rheumatologist in Knoxville, Tennessee, was the first to lay out diagnostic guidelines for fibromyalgia, classified as a disorder of pain processing due to abnormalities in how pain signals are processed in the central nervous system. The new (ICD-10) lists fibromyalgia as a diagnosable disease under "Diseases of the musculoskeletal system and connective tissue."

The Mayo Clinic states on their website that there are no known causes for fibromyalgia. Yet an investigational approach reveals that when looking at individuals with chronic widespread pain, a majority of them carry genetic glitches that may cause them to have a propensity to develop fibromyalgia. Why is it that some individuals with genetic polymorphisms *do not* develop the disease they have the mutation for? My personal theory is that toxins can permit these mutations to begin expressing. When a gene expresses itself, it permits the process of the disease to begin.

Once again, that silent killer black mold and mold toxicity may be an agent exacerbating fibromyalgia. Is it any wonder that I keep coming back to mold and other mycotoxins in these pages? By now you should see a pattern.

In my practice I find that many of my fibromyalgia patients have been exposed to mold. When we remove these toxins, the symptoms of fibromyalgia resolve. One particular patient had chronic headaches, muscle twitching, rapidity to the muscles, and excessive pain to the touch. After one week of treatment he could tolerate a massage, which then exasperated many symptoms. After three weeks of treatment his symptoms were 80 percent improved. Eventually he was able to go back to his regular work and begin to exercise again.

I have seen several women who, when optimized, were suddenly able to do tasks they never thought they were capable of—or hadn't done in many years. Some will lose weight after years of struggle, some can climb stairs again. I believe mold can be a real issue, but this is hard to control due to the additives in our food today, and even the traces of mold found in popular supplements.

The University of Maryland Medical Center suggests that environmental factors may also play a role in fibromyalgia, such as gasses from flooring, dry wall, carpet, insulations, and many other modern building components. Some physicians in independent medicine have noted that hormonal imbalances may also be part of the issue. Women may present with low progesterone levels, and when treated with bioidentical progesterone to near normal levels, the symptoms of fibromyalgia are often alleviated.

Other pathophysiology possibilities include dopamine, serotonin, neuroendocrine disruption, and sympathetic hyperactivity. All of these mechanisms must be taken into account when evaluating an individual with fibromyalgia.

As is so often the case with "mystery illnesses," I typically see that it is not just one component that needs optimizing, but multiple things. Fibromyalgia is very complex, much like Lyme disease. Due to subtle incongruences in many patients, all systems must be evaluated. For total healing balance, a full-spectrum treatment that encompasses amino acids, electrolytes, hormones, removing toxins, and lipid restoration must be done.

Next we'll take a look at fibromyalgia's close cousin—chronic fatigue—and how you can restore your health after years of this debilitating illness.

Chapter 7

Tired of Being Tired: Overcoming Chronic Fatigue and Adrenal Burnout

—⋙—

Also called adrenal fatigue by many in the integrated chiropractic and naturopathic world, chronic fatigue is a "malady of the modern age." With our world running at ever faster speeds, little to no downtime, stressors coming at us from all sides, poor diets, and a toxic environment, it's no surprise to me that so many people are afflicted with chronic fatigue. They limp into their doctor's offices, barely mustering the energy to crawl through their days, but often meet with a dismissive approach. Either it's "all in their heads" (the physician may say this is a kinder way) or they just need to boost their iron intake and reduce the stress in their lives. Problem solved, right?

While chronic fatigue sufferers may indeed need to reduce stress and increase their iron intake, I've found that it's rarely this simple. Adrenal fatigue, or adrenal burnout, is a complex issue—not a true ICD-10 diagnosis, but rather adrenal insufficiency and hypo-function of the adrenal glands. However, chronic fatigue does have an ICD-10. (ICD 9 and 10 are diagnoses laid out and accepted by insurance companies as well as by Medicare and Medicaid.)

This becomes a big dilemma due to the fact that two major different diseases or dysfunctions are at work here. Chronic fatigue is usually diagnosed only by relapsing fevers as well as intermittent lymph gland swelling. The individual may also have a sore throat. This invariably sounds like an infection of some sort. In these particular individuals I have found the Epstein-Barr virus, relapsing infections, and at times other parasite infections.

To complicate things, the symptoms of chronic fatigue often go along with fibromyalgia. Due to the relapsing nature of the symptoms, the diagnosis over time is usually difficult. For instance, Epstein-Barr is often present in other diseases such as Lyme and other co-infections.

Half of Us Are Exhausted
Moving on to adrenal fatigue, which is much more common, it is estimated that about 50 percent of the population has had adrenal fatigue at some

point. This is amazing when it is not even recognized by the regular medical community.

According to Wikipedia, adrenal fatigue or hypoadrenia are terms used in alternative medicine to describe the unscientific belief that the adrenal glands are exhausted and unable to produce adequate quantities of hormones, primarily the glucocorticoid cortisol. Adrenal fatigue should not be confused with recognized forms of adrenal dysfunction, such as adrenal sufficiency or Addison's disease.

The term "adrenal fatigue" was first described in 1998 by Dr. James M. Wilson, who went on to write a book labeling this malady "the 21st-century stress syndrome." Adrenal fatigue as a term is applied to mostly nonspecific symptoms. The salivary and urine tests done to diagnose adrenal fatigue are not accepted as scientific proof by the regular medical community. At one point the situation got so out of hand it resembled a lynch mob trying to remove medical licenses from physicians who believed after seeing countless patients that adrenal fatigue really does exist.

Common symptoms of adrenal fatigue include feeling tired for no reason, trouble waking up in the morning, even if you've had adequate sleep. So you need extra coffee or other stimulants in the morning if you feel rundown or overwhelmed. Other subtle symptoms are difficulty bouncing back after stress or illness and a craving for salty and sweet snacks. Some individuals with adrenal fatigue may feel more awake and energetic after 6 p.m. rather than earlier in the day.

You can see these are rather vague symptoms in the overall scheme of things. However, I have realized that most individuals with chronic illness or those taking care of the chronically ill will have adrenal fatigue.

What Causes Adrenal Fatigue (Hypoadrenia)?

The number one cause of adrenal fatigue is stress, and specifically stress that is related to grief or loss of some type. Some individuals who are in very stressful jobs with constant long hours and severe stress day after day will develop hypoadrenia. A body that is full of inflammation from illness, diet, and other factors will often attack the small adrenal glands sitting on top of the kidneys.

Even poor diet may lead to adrenal fatigue. Our bodies require specific foods for the production of glucocorticoids, and some foods not only work against this normal function but are highly inflammatory to the body—in particular sugary sweets, one of the highest inflammatory foods known to man. Diet is important as a preventative of adrenal fatigue and for the healing of adrenal fatigue as well as many other diseases. Although fasting may be good to eliminate toxins and cleanse the body, ironically, fasting is one of the *worst* things to do when fighting some chronic illness including adrenal fatigue.

Adrenal Fatigue's Three Stages

Most integrative physicians recognize three stages to adrenal fatigue. And although most know how to diagnose now through saliva or urine tests, the majority of these doctors still don't have the basics down for overall healing of the adrenals.

Stage 1: The first of the three stages is adrenal fatigue followed by high cortisol levels. When an individual is in stage one long enough the adrenals begin to burn out and stage two begins.

Stage 2: Stage two is marked by the falling of the cortisol. When random cortisol levels are tested, stage two may be missed because it may look normal. Stage two is when most individuals will begin to gain weight, have sleep disturbances, and lose their sex drive. When stage two is not addressed by changing diet, getting proper rest, and exercising appropriately, the individual progresses to stage three.

Let me make an important note here: some people with adrenal fatigue will overdo exercise, causing more stress on the adrenals. Cross-fit and long-distance running are examples of too strenuous a form of exercise. Short spurts of intense exercise are the best at permitting adequate time for the body to recover.

Stage 3: The last stage of adrenal fatigue is constant low cortisol levels, low and flat-lined. A person at this stage will not maintain a response to anything and will be tired all the time. They cannot get up and be motivated for work. They fall asleep at the wheel or at work. Sleep is just not refreshing. As already noted, they have a constant uncontrollable drive for salty foods alternating with sweet foods. Too many carbs continue to disrupt the cortisols.

Eventually this person will have blood pressure issues as well as a poor BP response to changing positions (known as POTS—postural orthostatic tachycardia syndrome). Gut immunity also becomes an issue as secretory IGA is regulated by cortisol. Therefore many individuals with gut issues may have abnormal levels of cortisol. This in turn affects every aspect of their bodies.

I have always believed we cannot compartmentalize our bodies. Each part affects the others. It is amazing how one small gland called the adrenals can affect so many parts of the body.

Adrenal Healing and Repair

Healing the adrenals takes six months to two years, and you must see a physician who actually knows how to treat this. Unfortunately, some doctors will simply push cortisone at patients, but this is one of the worst things you can do. I have had patients come in demanding cortisone because they were told they were going to die due to adrenal fatigue (this is all a false notion). Giving cortisone to adrenal fatigue only pushes down more of the cortisol produced by the adrenal gland.

The proper way to treat adrenal fatigue is by checking anti-inflammatory hormones and the mother of all hormones, pregnenolone. DHEA and pregnenolone are two major "ingredients" needed for adrenal healing and repair. Also needed are minerals and electrolytes. Changing this along with diet, rest, and proper exercise will permit slow natural healing over time. This approach, armed with knowing your fatty acid profile and which fats are needed as well as methylation pathways, enables health and healing. I have developed IV treatments that will shorten the healing by months.

An Overview of Adrenal Function

Your body's endocrine system is a delicately balanced yet powerful engine for energy production and an overall state of well-being. Here are the key players:

Adrenal glands – Two triangular-shaped glands that sit on top of your kidneys. They produce and secrete epinephrine (adrenaline, a fast-acting hormone), norepinephrine (noradrenaline), and a small amount of dopamine in response to stimulation by sympathetic preganglionic neurons. The adrenal cortex mediates the stress response through the production of steroid hormones, including cortisol, as well as DHEA and sex hormone precursors. **Cortisol** – The hormone released in response to any kind of stress. Its primary functions are to increase blood sugar; suppress the immune system; and aid in fat, protein, and carbohydrate metabolism. (Wiki)

Hypothalamus-Pituitary-Adrenal Axis (HPA Axis) – The system of communication between the neuro-endocrine glands that dictates our responses to stress as well as our circadian rhythm.[8]

Neurotransmitters – The chemical messengers that transmit signals from neurons to their target cells across synapses. The way each neurotransmitter is classified is based upon which receptors they activate.

Hippocampus and Circadian Rhythm – The gland that regulates circadian rhythm, our bodies' roughly twenty-four-hour cycle in biochemical, physiological, and behavioral processes.

When the neuro-endocrine pathways are well balanced, our bodies respond as they should—including a normal "fight or flight" reaction to episodes of stress, then returning to a relaxed state. But with prolonged or even chronic stress, we may experience acute bouts of an imbalance. Our bodies respond to the perceived fight or flight by pumping out more cortisol, but over time this constant flood of cortisol can be very damaging to our system. When stress becomes a way of life, the balance is lost and our bodies produce distress signals, often in the form of the ailments featured in this book.

Chronic Stress Wreaks Havoc on Your System

A typical stress response might occur when we are stuck in a traffic jam while on our way to an important meeting. But realize that similar stressors can affect different people in different ways, depending on their constitution as well as their mental, emotional, and physical well-being at the time the stressful event happens.

For example, two people may be in the same traffic jam, but one is perfectly happy to sit and listen to music on his iPod for an extra twenty minutes, while the other is about to be late for an important job interview. "The chain of events that happens in reaction to the traffic jam in each person's system will be very different as a result. Additionally, this response can be happening on a systemic level on a daily basis if you are eating food that you don't tolerate — *your weekly gluten-bomb cheats that you think aren't so bad ... they are.* And your body is trying to recover from the inflammation in your gut without reprieve."[9]

A pattern of repeated excitatory response, or even chronic internal stress such as malnutrition or gut irritation, can push your immuno-endocrine system completely off balance. Now you see how critical proper nutrition, adequate exercise, gut health, and positive thoughts, emotions, perceptions, and reactions to life stressors really are in keeping the adrenal glands in check.

The single biggest contributing factor to adrenal fatigue is stress. We live in an incredibly stressful world of "need it yesterday" deadlines, road rage, and accelerated everything—literally, the pace of everything is sped up when we compare it to how people lived just half a century ago. Go back a century or more, and you can see how alarmingly fast our world spins today.

But we can't just stop our lives, so what do we do? It's impossible to avoid stress altogether. Instead, we must identify the forms that we can best control in our lives and work on making diet and lifestyle modifications to lower the stress-load on our systems.

Contributors to the stress that leads to adrenal fatigue can be lifestyle stressors including:

- lack of sleep
- poor food choices
- use of stimulants
- pulling all-nighter or pushing through a day despite being tired
- perfectionism
- staying in no-win situations for too long
- over-training
- lack of fun or stress-relieving practices[10]

High-pressure jobs, intense school work, being in unhappy marriages or miserable jobs, feeling overall dissatisfaction with your life—all these and other factors can lead to adrenal fatigue. Life events can also lead to hypoadrenia. These may include a crisis or severe emotional trauma, the death of a loved one, major surgery, extended or chronic illness, and sudden change in your life situation (e.g. loss of a job).

While adrenal fatigue can sabotage us suddenly when triggered by a traumatic life event, more often it is the result of a gradual, cumulative effect of multiple stressors.

We can bring our adrenal health back in balance through managing the stressors in our life and (you guessed it) getting our glutathione levels back to optimum levels. On a practical, day-to-day basis, here are some things you can do:

- Sleep
- Avoid draining people or situations (learn to say NO to things!)
- Do not over-train
- Do restorative exercises (meditation, restorative breathing, walking, light yoga)
- Whenever you are not enjoying your life, assess whether you can
  change the situation
  change yourself to fit the situation
  leave the situation

- Keep a gratitude list
- Play (with family, friends, pets)[11]

Chapter 8

"It Was Just a Tick Bite"— Lyme: The Silent Killer

—∭—

The first time I saw Gary, his father carried him in. Only forty-nine years old, he was completely weak and wasted, with a hollow look to his eyes. Gary's skin had a grayish cast, and I learned that he had been homebound and bedbound for two years at this point. In search of a cure, Gary had seen some elite doctors in the United States, doctors who diagnosed and treated him for Lyme disease, adrenal fatigue, and chronic candidiasis.

After all these treatments Gary was only getting worse. He had occasional seizures—a new and puzzling addition to the list of symptoms. As the years of failed treatments wore on, Gary, like many chronically ill patients, sensed a growing frustration and rejection by his parents and friends. People get tired of hearing how sick they are and label them hypochondriacs; siblings get upset because the sick person is draining the parents' inheritance, time, and emotions. The emotional strain exacted a heavy toll on Gary—so much so that he spent time in a psychiatric ward.

Lyme disease is caused by the bacterium Borrelia burgdorferi, and is transmitted to humans through the bite of infected blacklegged ticks. Often the infected person doesn't even know they got bitten by a tick. Maybe they played near the woods as a child or went on camping trips with a scouting troop. The early symptoms of Lyme—fever, head-ache, fatigue, and skin rash—can easily be mistaken for a common cold or other bug. If left untreated, however, infection can spread to joints, the heart, and eventually the nervous system.

So here was a man with extreme confusion and clinical aloofness, estranged from everyone. He couldn't interact well, even with me. We started IV treatments and gave Gary a small amount of methionine (an amino acid); immediately he went into seizure. We reversed the seizure within seconds, but I knew I had to look deeper into his genetic profile—something was very wrong. After further study I realized Gary had a genetic glitch that caused him to be unable to tolerate methionine.

In his previous treatment for Lyme he had received excessive amounts of antibiotics, a treat-ment plan that I believe caused further DNA glitches and problems with his methylation pathways. Gary's chemical sensitivities were so strong he hadn't been in a restaurant for three years. If someone entered a room wearing perfume, his body immediately reacted.

After a deeper look at his genetic profile, I realized Gary was going to be a slow process because he had so many genetic glitches that he could not tolerate very much. So we took a slow and steady approach with him—administering IV therapy (essential fatty acids with some amino acids he could tolerate), glutathione supplements, other macronutrients/supplements, and dietary changes.

Over the course of a year he retained the ability to live on his own, and today he can walk a mile, drive a car, and interact normally again. He even wrote a book that won an award. The Gary I see today is more energetic and hopeful about his life. This doesn't mean he never has bad times—stress, for instance, can cause a relapse of his symptoms. But after eighteen years of being critically ill, he's on a path to improving every day.

I learned an important truth through my treatment of Gary: if you don't look at a person's genetics, you could be pushing them down a path of demise.

Tracing the History of Lyme Disease

Typically called a tick-borne illness, Lyme disease was first noted in children who all had the same symptoms, and all the symptoms were related to tick bites. These reoccurring set of symptoms included a telltale rash (erythema-migrans) at the site of the tick bite, what appeared to be juvenile onset rheumatoid arthritis, and severe fatigue. Usually these symptoms appeared in the summer and in children living near wooded areas. Due to these reccurring signs and symptoms it was given the name Lyme.

Later in 1981 the cause of Lyme was pinpointed to be Borrelia burdorferi, a spirochete in which the outer surface appeared like a gram-negative bacteria, but this was not a bacteria but a spirochete with flagella. These flagella enabled the spirochetes to hide themselves from the host's immune system.

When we look back in history we can see that Lyme symptoms were first reported in the 1600s. Also, science has proven that the Iceman—a Neolithic man frozen in ice 5,300 years ago—had Borrelia burdorferi DNA found in his frozen body. Apparently, this individual had Lyme disease, but we don't know if it was the cause of his demise or whether he died from something else.

Why, you may ask, am I telling you all these boring facts? Well, because they lay the groundwork for problems we encounter with Lyme disease. Currently there are three strains of Borrelia: Borrelia burdorferi, Borrelia aarnii, and Borrelia afzelii. The second two are not common in North America but are found in Europe and Asia.

Borrelia burdorferi has unique outer membrane proteins that proteins play a large role in the spirochete's virulence. And the flagella are normally antigenic from the host's immune defense—meaning they stimulate the production of an antibody in the body.

Because the spirochete is like a gram-negative bacteria in its cell membrane, it can put off exotoxins. Endotoxins and exotoxins can bind to specific receptors in the body and be highly antigenic. These toxins, in fact, play a large role in the Lyme symptoms. However, an individual's genetic makeup and epigenetic profile will offer a glimpse as to which areas of the body will be affected. The exotoxins from Lyme can be controlled by extra-chromosome genes. (The exotoxins and endotoxins from Lyme will cause the epigenetic profiles to either stop functioning or over function. This causes disregulation of our biological pathways.)

Genetics and epigenetics reveal areas where Lyme toxins can be lodged and affecting an individual. If this were not so, then why are there so many varying types of symptoms, and why is Lyme often called the "Great Imitator"? In layman's terms, epigenetics is the study of external or environmental factors that turn genes *on* and *off* and affect how cells *read* genes.[12]

Signs and Symptoms of Lyme
Many practitioners break them up into stages, as follows.

Stage One: Erythema-migrans. This is a rash at the site of a tick bite. However, I have met very few Lyme patients who ever had this symptom. Also in stage one are headaches or flu-like symptoms and stiff neck. A large number of people recall these symptoms, but some may have never had these symptoms at all.

Stage Two: Memory problems. The person may also have lower extremity weakness.

Stage Three: Swelling, pain, arthritis, and weakness of facial muscles, often misdiagnosed as Bell's palsy. Also occurring in this stage are numbness and tingling in your hands, feet, and/or back.

My treatment plan for Lyme includes discovering an individual's unique genetic profile. Then I develop a treatment plan specifically for that person. Most Lyme patients have large amounts of toxin buildup and need these toxins removed so that normal body function can be restored.

As someone who suffered from untreated Lyme disease for years, I can attest to how serious this disease is. The sad thing is that many conventional physicians will misdiagnose this illness, prescribing drugs for a battery of symptoms but missing the real culprit. In the story below, you'll meet a woman who came to me for treatment after decades of suffering from Lyme disease.

HELEN: "INTO THE WOODS"— AND OUT WITH A CHRONIC ILLNESS

Today I am forty-eight years old and live a healthy life. But it was not always that way. When I was twenty-three and still a young bride, my husband and I went camping after taking a break from remodeling our house. Camping in Yosemite National Forest was great and so beautiful, and I just could not believe the majesty of it all.

The morning before our last day I woke up with what appeared to be a bug bite on my leg. The bite had a puffiness and swelling around it. After about three days, it became very hot to the touch but had no rash or anything else to indicate the spreading of an infection. This went away, and six weeks later we participated in a 10k run. After my run I developed shortness of breath, vertigo, and constant nausea.

We continued working on our house but ran into a few problems and later found out it had had some flood damage in the past. Inexplicably, I began losing weight and the nausea was getting worse. I was now having problems of constipation with intermittent diarrhea. Concerned, I went to my doctor, who diagnosed me with IBS and told me to change my diet. After changing my diet I continued to lose weight.

My husband said I was no longer attractive and started having an affair with a coworker. Devastated by his betrayal, I moved back in with my parents and two weeks later my father had a stroke. Still I continued to lose weight. My mother took me to Emory and I was told that I had anorexia nervosa.

They kept me hospitalized but I continued to have all of my symptoms, but now I was vomiting and had even more diarrhea.

They started an IV with a PICC line for hyper alimentation. I did gain back about ten pounds in two and a half months, but overall my health was declining. Someone referred me to Dr. Crozier, and the test for Lyme came back negative, but he said I had CD57 that looks like Lyme; however, he could not diagnose me with Lyme on a CD57 alone. After further genetic testing, we discovered that I did have the Borrelia bacteria (Lyme) in my system. He also noted that I had labs indicating probable mold toxicity.

I suddenly realized I had been exposed to black mold while remodeling our home several years in a row, which was many years ago now. I had spent most of my life bedridden, going in and out of the hospital and getting many tests as well as IV hyper alimentation. This was getting very tiresome. At this point my mother had been my caretaker for about twenty years. She was exhausted and so was I.

Dr. Crozier recommended counseling for both my mother and me. We followed his recommendation and received a lot of benefit from it. He also gave me positive affirmations to say, and I read them on a daily basis—in fact my mother also began to say them. He started me on a regime to heal my body, mind, and spirit. As I began to have healing, my strength gradually came back. I gained weight and learned how to detox my body from mold, mycotoxins, heavy metals, pesticides, herbicides, and many other toxins.

Am I completely normal? No, but Dr. Crozier never guaranteed I would be back to a normal life. He told me he always believed in hope. I developed hope for the future. Now most of my life was past, or at least all the years women become mothers and are productive, and I felt ashamed, confused, and upset. I needed to deal with my feelings of being a failure and not being able to have the life I once dreamed for myself.

I continue to deal with these issues, but I can truly say that most are dealt with and I have hope for the future again. Even now I am thinking about dating again and perhaps having hope for a life mate one day. I wish someone would have told me years ago how deadly mold really is. Dr. Crozier revealed it was not just Lyme but Lyme and mold together that caused my issues. Yet, in spite of all that has happened to me, I have hope. We all can have hope.

Chapter 9

Look Who's Coming to Dinner: Getting Rid of Internal Parasites

—ɯ—

Two weeks before Thanksgiving in 2013, Kathy noticed a persistent itching in her rectal area. *I must have hemorrhoids*, she thought, dismissing the thought as soon as it came and making a mental note to pick up some Preparation H at the local pharmacy. But several days of application brought no relief. In fact, she was getting worse, with open sores that were itchy, swollen, and inflamed. Finally she went to her primary care physician to get help.

"I think I have hemorrhoids, but please don't touch me because it hurts really bad," she told her doctor, who examined her and "looked like he had fear in his eyes." He told Kathy he didn't know what was wrong with her, but he gave her a prescription for yeast infection, told her to eat more fiber, and recommended she see a colorectal surgeon. Having completed the appointment, he "practically ran out of the room," she remembers.

"I didn't have any manifestations of parasites yet," says Kathy, "but I think they were trying to lay eggs in me. Dr. Crozier later told me it was possibly from something I ate, maybe in a restaurant, and they went to that area and were incubating. Cockroaches, for example, carry other parasites."

The colorectal surgeon inserted a scope to investigate but couldn't see anything. After taking a stool sample, he told Kathy she most likely had pinworms. She knew she didn't have pinworms because they're visible, and he never saw anything. After the stool sample, he too told her he didn't know what was wrong with her, so he sent her to an infectious disease specialist.

By this time her husband, Alan, had caught whatever strange infestation was attacking Kathy. Now she had horrendous bursts of swarming all over her vaginal area—though the "critters" were still too small to be seen.

"It felt like thousands were crawling all over me," she says. "The infectious disease specialist gave me terrible advice. She said, 'Go home, love each other, hug your grandchildren, and sleep with your husband.' At this point we had separated from our children and grandchildren to protect them from whatever was in our house. The specialist thought Alan was being sympathetically ill. She just told us to enjoy life and smile. We were furious."

At one point Kathy and Alan considered going to Johns Hopkins for answers, but when Alan told the intake staff what they were dealing with, they informed him the treatment would include four to six weeks of psychotherapy before any other treatment program could begin. "I knew we weren't nuts," he said. "We didn't bother going."

By now Kathy was starting to have visible bites from the nightly swarms. Alan moved into their guestroom to try to avoid infestation.

"The bugs would wake me up and crawl all over my face," Kathy says. "It felt like they were trying to get in my eyelids, go up my nose; they even filled up my navel once they became of a size that I could see. When I had a bowel movement my stool was loaded with stuff—little white balls that looked like eggs. Then I had bugs that were large—the size of two raisins stuck together. One time I passed a large creature that looked like something prehistoric with no coating on it, and no skeleton. I never showed Alan because it was so horrifying. We were now in a panic stage and were felt like we were literally being eaten alive. There were blood dots all over us. Alan's entire back was bug-bitten. I had bug bites covering my private areas."

Spraying Lysol on everything gave a little relief, and it reached the point where Kathy was spraying herself with Lysol. Alan hired people to come in and tent their house for three days. "But we were contagious so where could we go?" says Kathy. "We had to go to a hotel but were terrified that we could pass it to someone else. We would stay just one night, then spray the carpets and bedding, and rip everything up so they would wash everything."

Desperate for answers, Alan started searching online for someone who knew about parasites. They realized they couldn't tell anybody in their social circle; it was too private, too embarrassing— and the doctors didn't believe them.

In the end, they heard about me through a seminar at our church. With nothing else to lose, they came to me for a consultation and told me the story you're reading here.

Alan: With Dr. Crozier, we learned something very quickly. Other doctors will send you to a standard lab to get a blood workup. But we were dealing with a micro-infestation in our bodies, and a standard lab can't test to the level where these creatures live. I was told there are only two or three labs in entire country that have this type of microscopic viewing. When the blood samples came back, Kathy had six or more different types of parasites living in her body, expanding and growing. The normal medical process could not have found this.

Kathy: With the right lab work, I could have proved to the naysayer doctors that I wasn't crazy because now I had pictures. With 400x magnification, you can see them. Alan was so thin and weak at this point, but he cut up all the carpet by himself and hauled it out to be destroyed. We couldn't let

---

anyone in the house. The bugs were everywhere. If I washed the counter down, there were little black dots—and they move very quickly throughout your home.

By reading online we learned that we could tape off parts of our house, trying to lessen the movement of the bugs. Alan cut open our mattress and there they were. We sliced open his recliner and there they were. I was so traumatized.

I couldn't sleep at night because I was being eaten, so I figured out that if you placed duct tape over the anus, blocking up your outlet there, the bugs couldn't get out. Alan would cut duct tape every night and seal up that area so the bugs couldn't get out. I got so much relief and could finally rest at night.

Alan: In February 2014, I finally called Dr. Crozier. It was late afternoon on a Friday, and I thought, *It's Friday … nobody will answer.* But his wife, Michelle, answered and I told her our story. "I want the whole story," she said. Ten minutes later Dr. Crozier came on the line and we did a three-way call. "I know what's wrong with you," he said. "I want you in here on Monday morning." And so we made our appointment.

Kathy: Dr. Crozier showed such compassion and concern for us, it almost brought us to tears, because nobody had cared—and many thought we had mental illness. He gave me intravenous vitamin C followed by a series of IVs with amino acids, hydrogen peroxide, and other things. He took our blood and got proof that the parasites were in my blood. I had actually saved a bunch of the bugs I could see, and he said he had never seen so many varieties inside one person.

So we'd go to his office every week and have these treatments. He also put us on several supplements, including one called "blue clay"—literally blue clay in a capsule. You take the capsules, drink water, then soak in a hot tub, and the bugs come out. I saw things that looked like pollywogs, long snaky things a quarter-inch long, black dots, little round things. Sometimes there would be twenty or thirty of them, but as time went on there were fewer and fewer. We did these soaks every single night for months.

Dr. Crozier was our salvation. Nobody else wanted to see us. He worked with us, was patient with us, and would change our treatment plan if he felt like we needed something different. After the treatment program he did another blood workup on us. By my second blood test he believed the infestation was about 85 percent controlled.

Our house is now clean. Yes, we are still battling parasites in our skin that are so strong they're just hanging on. But we're wearing them down through a new treatment paradigm to get rid of them once and for all. I thank God for sending a shining light to us in a sea of fear.

A Parallel Universe

Many people may think, *Oh, this does not apply to me—I could never have parasites living inside my body.* But wait! Let's list the common symptoms that could possibly be signs of parasites before you ignore this. These parasites are far more common than you might think. You may be scrupulously clean, live in an upscale neighborhood, never travel to third-world countries, and still contract parasites.

The stigma associated with parasite infestation points a finger of blame, implying that the affected persons are dirty and have poor hygiene; the story of Alan and Kathy shows that *anyone* can contract these bugs, regardless of their lifestyle.

Here are a few common signs and symptoms of parasite infections:

- IBS, diarrhea leading to constipation, gas, and bloating; sometimes feeling things moving in the abdomen
- History of food poisoning and knowing your digestion has never been the same since
- Eczema, hives, rashes, and other skin irritations (I have literally seen parasites crawl out from an individual's skin)
- Sleep difficulties that can range from trouble falling asleep to waking up multiple times during the night
- Grinding your teeth if not caused by something else that can be explained
- Burning under the scalp
- Joint aches and pains, muscle spasms
- Fatigue, depression, and severe exhaustion

- Unsatisfied appetite—never feeling satisfied after meals
- Unexplained weight loss
- Unexplained anemia

What Exactly Are Parasites?

A parasite is an organism that lives in and off of another organism, called a host. Think of fleas and ticks and heartworms afflicting a dog. In this case, the host is the dog and the parasites literally make a meal of the dog. Unfortunately, parasites target humans too. Parasites are dependent upon the host for survival—the ability to live, grow, and multiply. They cannot live independently. Parasites very rarely kill their host but can do so in some cases.

The word "parasite" comes from the Greek word *parasites—para* meaning alongside and *sitos* meaning food. Prior to the eighteenth century, the word parasite was used to describe family or friends who overstayed their welcome, or one who was living off the expenses of another person. After the eighteenth century, it became a biological term. There are three main types of parasites.

1. Protozoa—a single-cell organism; one example is malaria. Protozoa can only multiply inside of a host cell.

2. Helminths—examples include roundworm, pinworm, trichina, spiralis, fluke, and tapeworm
3. Anthropods—insects that carry parasites

Although you may contract a parasite in a number of ways, the most common way is through contaminated food and/or water. Foods imported from third-world countries are high-risk for parasites because many of these countries use human feces to fertilize the foods, increasing the likelihood of passing eggs, cysts, or parasites themselves to many others.

Lakes, ponds, and creeks can all contain parasites. When we were kids, many of us swam in natural lakes or ponds, and our parents would pour hydrogen peroxide in our ears afterward to cut our risk of infestation. Undercooked meats may also contain eggs and parasites, as well as contaminated fruits and vegetables.

If a person has been infected, the parasites can easily spread to the handles on the sink faucet, door handles in restrooms, and saltshakers in a restaurant. Parasites have even been found on an infected person's cell phone. Touching or handling any of these and then touching your eyes, nose, or mouth is an easy way to become contaminated with various types of parasites.

Some individuals will not even know they have become contaminated and may in fact be contaminating others. This is the reason I am seeing growing numbers of patients contaminated and becoming extremely ill from massive parasite infections. In my clinic, the numbers are increasing weekly of those suffering from symptoms that are going undiagnosed in the traditional medical community—and it is parasites causing these unbelievable problems for the patients.

Typically you think of diarrhea as a symptom of parasitic invasion, but more often I am seeing constipation as a real problem. Another common symptom is muscle pain unexplained by other physicians, which could be due to water content in the bowel and the body changing.

Targeting the Bugs

How do we test for these parasites? In the past we only did the conventional stool analysis testing, which can still be done. This analysis tests for parasites and parasite eggs and requires three separate stools to analyze under a microscope. The pathologist needs to be proficient at identifying these parasites or ova (eggs). What happens if the parasites are dormant at the time of testing, or not even living in the gut but in the bloodstream or brain? If either of those scenarios occurs, an individual can have a false negative result.

Today more doctors are changing to stool tests that use PCR (polymerase chain reaction) technology. This test amplifies the parasite's DNA, so it can be dormant or alive and still be detected. PCR can identify up to seventeen different types of parasites.

If the parasite is only in the brain, it is very difficult to identify when they become advanced to an aggressive state. However, parasites in the brain may be seen by an MRI. I have had several patients whose MRIs revealed spirochetes in the brain, most likely from Lyme. A simple blood test may reveal an enlarged RDW (red cell distribution width). This does not always mean intracellular parasites, but it can be at many times.

The study and treatment of parasites is a growing field, and we must continue to look for more advanced ways of testing for parasites due to the fact that these bugs are exploding in our society.

Treating parasites depends on the location and type. Traditionally we had Biltricide, Ivermectin, Pyrantel Pamoate, Albenza, and Alinia. I still use these medications but have found them incomplete or too harsh for some of my patients. Often I will combine homeopathic and sometimes a blend of herbs, including grapefruit. These are often tolerated well and can help rid a patient of parasites.

One mineceutical (an antibacterial K-rectorite blue clay-based mineral) studied by Arizona State University was found to be effective in getting parasites, candida, and other bugs under control. This can't be used for extensive amounts of time due to high iron levels. Each person must be treated individually as they need and require.

At Excellent Living, some individuals require extensive IV treatment along with oral treatment. Treatment can get very difficult when you suddenly realize there are now more parasites than we are even able to test for.

Eating for Life

I believe diet is a crucial part of treatment in all aspects of health. I try to individualize diets according to a person's genetics. Can they tolerate high-sulfur foods or not? Can they tolerate meat, or should they be on a low-meat diet? However, *everyone* needs to be off sugar. It's a high-inflammatory food. And everyone needs to consume vegetables and berries. Berries are low glycemic and tolerated by most.

Many of my patients have had severe problems at night when the parasites began to move and migrate. Some will get severe insomnia and almost have the need for a psychiatric visit. I have had several who experienced night tremors with sweating, scalp burning, and even feelings of going insane! When bugs are crawling on you or in you, your sanity may be holding on by a mere thread. The psychological implications are unbelievable. Antipsychotics are of little benefit with these parasites.

Once again I have to turn to genetics because what I have seen is that individuals contaminated with parasites have epigenetic changes affecting the "Gads"—RS1050828, GAD1, and many more. My personal belief is that these parasites and the toxins from killing the parasites get lodged in the areas where we have genetic mutations. These areas are weak and vulnerable to toxins, and the intruders causing them begin to express and reveal symptoms. These symptoms will preclude many practitioners from finding the real cause, which in the long run will break down the person's body.

Let us live well, heal our cells, and get rid of the harmful parasites that can make our very existence difficult to deal with.

Chapter 10

Life Off-Kilter:
Addressing Hormonal Imbalance

—⟋⟍—

Some celebrities have made the topic of hormones, and staying "forever young," very popular. Recognizing a groundswell, the anti-aging doctors got on the bandwagon of hormones and bioidentical hormones too. Personally I have known the benefits of hormones for many years as a practicing OB/GYN before I left the field to go into integrative medicine, treating the difficult cases most traditional doctors have given up on.

While working as an OB/GYN we were taught the basics about hormones. However, after being in and going to many courses offered by the American Academy of Anti-Aging Medicine (A4M) on bioidentical hormones and hormone replacement, I suddenly realized that hormones for women and men were much more involved than what I thought.

One key revelation was that estrogen has many more positive effects than just helping to prevent hot flashes. Estrogen has a significant health benefit on brain tissue, and the same is true with progesterone. In my practice I found that testosterone had much more of an effect than just increasing libido—in fact it helps with our immune system as well.

Progesterone: Friend or Foe?

Lately there has been much controversy over supplementing with progesterone and estradiol. Some have even demonized these hormones. Why? Because certain studies[13] show an increased risk of breast cancer for individuals who take these two hormones, as compared to taking estrogen alone. However, these clinical trials were done on synthetic progestins. This is troublesome due to the fact that other studies have shown no increased risk for breast cancer with pulsed natural progesterone from a bioidentical source. The studies showing that there is no increase in cancer with bioidentical hormones are continually pushed down or brushed to the side, declared as not credible by other experts in the field. Like all studies, some are more credible than others.

The benefits of progesterone are:

- Maintains uterine lining and prevents excess buildup
- Inhibits breast tissue overgrowth

- Increases metabolism and promotes weight loss
- Balances blood sugar levels
- Acts as a natural diuretic
- Normalizes blood clotting
- Stimulates the production of new bone
- Enhances the action of thyroid hormones
- Alleviates depression and anxiety
- Promotes normal sleeping patterns
- Prevents or manages cyclical migraines
- Restores proper cell oxygen levels
- Improves libido

Some common symptoms of progesterone deficiency are:

- Irritability
- Hypersensitivity
- Nervousness
- Restless sleep
- Headaches/ migraines before menstruation
- Weight gain
- Breast tenderness
- Decreased libido
- Heavy periods

Natural progesterone was discovered in the 1930s by Professor Russell Marker of Pennsylvania State University. His research brought natural progesterone from wild yams, often called

micronized progesterone or bioidentical progesterone. This form of progesterone is processed by
the human body and recognized as being the same
as what the body produces.

Natural and synthetic progesterone are not
molecularly identical. The synthetic forms are
called progestins and are very potent. Some forms
of progestins, such as medroxy progesterone, are
linked to blood clots, fluid retention, acne, weight
gain instead of weight loss, depression, and rashes.
These progestins are able to bind to glucocorticoids
and mineral corticoid receptors in the body. This
explains the wide range of side effects many woman
experience while taking progestins. While progesterone has many effects on the body, it also has up
to four hundred different beneficial functions.

More Than a Libido Booster
Estrogen also has a multitude of effects, with over
four hundred functions. These include much more
than just some libido issues (that benefit seems
to get everyone's attention!). Just to put it out like
this, the common myth is that estrogen is needed
by both women and men.

What are some of the commonly known benefits of estrogen?

- Encourages uterine lining growth
- Inhibits FSH (follicle-stimulating hormone)
  production

- Stimulates the pituitary gland
- Inhibits LH (luteinizing hormone) after ovulation
- Stimulates egg release (causing only one egg to mature)
- Helps maintain body temperature (woman and men)
- Delays memory loss
- Increases serotonin
- Protects nerves from damage
- Improves collagen
- Increases skin thickness
- Improves blood supply

Estrogen positively impacts the following areas of the body:

- Adrenal cortex
- Placenta
- Liver
- Breasts
- Fat cells
- Male testes
- Brain tissue for neuro-receptors

Those are only a few things that can be affected by estrogen.

The Downside: Risks of Estrogen

Prominent European studies[14]) showed a difference between bioidentical and synthetic progesterone in that the *synthetic progesterone* had the following risks:

- Heart attack
- Stroke
- Blood clots
- Pulmonary embolism
- Nausea
- Vomiting
- Headaches
- Weight gain
- Breast tenderness
- Increased breast size

Estrogen, in proper quantities and bioidentical form, has more safety than using the potent synthetic estrogens. Estrogen may help:

- Decrease hot flashes
- Improve moods
- Improve sleep
- Reduce vaginal irritation
- Reduce osteoporosis
- Reduce risk of dental problems including gum disease
- Improve vaginal dryness
- Lesson anxiety

- Improve libido (for women)
- Improve cholesterol metabolism

A Male Menopause?

Recent studies are showing that just as women have menopause, men also experience a dramatic decrease in testosterone production in the middle-age years, causing changes in sexual function and body composition. We have some results in the following diseases related to estrogen—either too little or too much, or receiving endogenous estrogen or incorrect types or amounts. Some of these have no estrogen (men just like women can have too little or too much estrogen):

- Breast cancer
- Endometrial cancer
- Ovarian cancer
- Colorectal cancer
- Heart disease
- Alzheimer's
- Parkinson's
- Gallbladder
- Osteoporosis
- Lupus and other autoimmune diseases

Benefits of the Big T

Testosterone gets a lot of press for starting wars and causing road rage, but it's not just a "male" hormone. Like estrogen, it too is also very important for both men and women. As with the previous hormones discussed, the benefits of testosterone cover much more than just the libido.

Testosterone affects the:

- Libido
- Hypothalamus
- Pituitary-sending signal
- Behavioral traits (confidence)
- Central nervous system
- Muscle mass
- Bone density
- Fat metabolism
- Heart health
- Skin repair
- Sperm production

So what are some possible signs and symptoms of testosterone deprivation?

- Depression
- Muscle loss/ muscle wasting
- Cognitive decline
- Lack of self-confidence
- Hair loss
- Increased central obesity (fat around the middle section)
- Loss of libido
- Fatigue
- Lack of motivation

• Bone loss/ osteoporosis

Pregnenolone: The Mother of All Hormones

A natural cascading of hormones occurs as we age, and the mother of all hormones which starts the cascade is pregnenolone. One major problem is that now we are lowering cholesterol to such low states that we convert very little cholesterol to pregnenolone. Our bodies try to make up the difference by producing more cholesterol to overcome the low levels of hormones we need for optimal function.

Pregnenolone has been shown in studies to be very significant for cognitive functioning. Adequate levels of this hormone heal the neuro-steroids and neuro-active-steroids. These very small yet complex molecules act in similar ways to neurotransmitters.

Normalizing levels of pregnenolone and neuro-steroids in the brain promotes neurogenesis, or the production of new nerve cells. It also helps with normal survival myelination (demyelinization is associated with multiple sclerosis and other neurological diseases), increased memory, and reduced neurotoxicity. Unfortunately, neurotoxicity affects all individuals in this day and age. Balancing hormones is part of the process for cell healing and repair. Science will continue to delve into deeper, more current research in this area to permit continued healing one cell at a time.

What About Steroids?

Once again, here's a topic that has been blown up by the media due to celebrity athlete abuse of steroids to grow preternatural muscle mass or increase speed, but that doesn't mean we should "throw the baby out with the bathwater" as the old saying goes.

Steroids are a large family of structurally similar biochemicals that have sex-determining, anti-inflammatory, and growth-regulatory roles. Indeed, pregnenolone is the grand precursor from which almost all the other steroid hormones are made: including DHEA, progesterone, testosterone, the estrogens, and cortisol. Despite its powerful metabolites, pregnenolone is acknowledged to be without significant side effects, with minimal or no anabolic, estrogenic, or androgenic activity. In other words, it will not cause too much estrogen or testosterone in the body.

Other benefits of pregnenolone may include stress reduction and increased resistance to the effects of stress, improvement of mood and energy, reduced symptoms of PMS and menopause, improved immunity, and repair of myelin sheaths—the insulating layer that forms around nerves and facilitates the transmission of nerve impulses. Pregnenolone also operates as a powerful neurosteroid in the brain, modulating the transmission of messages from neuron to neuron and strongly influencing learning and memory processes. As with

DHEA, pregnenolone levels naturally peak during youth and begin a long, slow decline with age.

With almost all diseases there appears to be an imbalance of hormones, and I therefore test each individual for hormones. In my treatment plan I will optimize hormones to aid in the body's ability to heal itself. I have noticed that as the body heals, most individuals can be weaned off all bio-identical hormones and will need nothing once the body is functioning in a normal capacity.

You're How Old?—Hormones for Anti-Aging

As the Baby Boomers continue to age, I expect to see more and more people turning to hormone replacement therapy and other natural remedies to the aging process. As of this writing, I am fifty-seven years old and yet people almost always think I'm fifteen to twenty years younger.

It would benefit no one if I preached a Fountain of Youth gospel but looked tired and wasted and old beyond my years. Even though my childhood hit me with a debilitating illness (Lyme disease), the subsequent years of combating that damage through proper eating, the right supplemental daily "cocktail," and overall healthy living have restored my natural vitality—with the added benefit of a youthful appearance.

There is no such thing as "anti-aging" without being whole from the inside out. You can have your cellulite siphoned out through liposuction, your body nipped and tucked, but if your under-lying foundation—the cellular you—is sick or weak, that damage will show through accelerated aging, period.

Have you ever seen an older woman with a face stretched so tight it gave her a death-grimace instead of a natural smile? She may have been trying desperately, through plastic surgery, to turn back the clock, but all you see is an old woman with oddly tight skin—not a naturally youthful-looking woman whose real age defies the birth date on her driver's license.

In our quest to stay young and young looking for as long as possible, we can't do any better than to start healing our bodies from the inside out ... one cell at a time.

And that's the topic of our next chapter.

Chapter 11
Prevention Is the Best
Anti-Aging 'Medicine'

—⟳—

Anti-aging has become a $50 billion industry just in the United States alone.

One day at lunch I overheard a conversation at the next table and became quite interested. The people talking appeared to be between forty-five and fifty-five years of age. They were talking about how they used to travel and do all these hiking trips and other things in the '70s—lamenting that they really didn't have the ability to do the things they used to do anymore.

I suddenly started thinking of myself and friends that I graduated with. These friends now look much older than I do, and I was the one who had gotten sick and prior could not even do as much as some of my closest friends could do.

As our society ages and this becomes a problem, it will exact a devastating toll on our communities.

Production will fall, gross national production will drop. With so many individuals who are currently able to produce becoming sick and older, and suddenly not able to perform the same functions, our entire societal infrastructure will wobble. For the Baby Boomers, that generation who felt they would stay "forever young," old age is a scary new reality looming on the horizon. And that horizon is getting closer and closer with every passing day.

Inner—Not Just Outer—Health

Unfortunately, in today's society we are more interested in outer appearances rather than the inner health that means the most. Yet our inner health and healing have a profound effect on our outer looks. I have seen time and time again that when we begin the agents that will halt and sometimes reverse aging, we start to look and feel much younger. Youth is something every single person tries to attain. We especially try to hold onto the aspect of youth and young living in our older age.

More than any other area in alternative health, anti-aging is guilty of promising magic-bullet fixes from miracle wrinkle-reducing creams to human growth hormone supplements. It's no wonder the market is growing exponentially.

But there is no magic bullet. The simple fact is that aging is not the result of any one single factor, but the cumulative result of a number of factors, including:

- Cell senescence, or the aging of cells
- Diminished telomerase activity
- Protein degradation
- Advanced glycation end products
- Excess sugar activity
- Progressive systemic inflammation
- Progressive dehydration
- Accumulated toxic build-up in organ tissue
- Reduced circulation
- Reduced cellular energy production
- Changes in hormone levels and hormone balance
- Impeded energy flows in the body
- Excessive body weight
- Old-fashioned wear and tear[15]

Add to this list the effects of stress, poor diet, mycotoxins, and the accumulation of free radicals in the body. Taken altogether, they create a perfect storm of accelerated aging. Some individuals age faster depending on their genetics and how well they can detoxify. For those who cannot detoxify on their own (due to the HLA-DRBQ genetic glitch), the result is massive amounts of toxins accumulating in their cells, causing excess aging.

In his article "The Nature of Aging," Jon Barron states, "If you want to slow the aging process, you have to look at more than a magic bullet approach involving one or two supplements. The only way to maximize health and lifespan is to use a Baseline of Health® type whole-body systemic approach. In other words, you need to do everything all at once."[16]

Don't be overwhelmed by that statement. Through a series of proactive steps on your part, you can slow or even reverse the aging process and stay more youthful, vibrant, and energized for longer than you ever thought possible.

What Can You Do to Turn Back the Clock?

- Rebuild liver function
- Lose weight
- Flush toxins
- Reduce caloric intake
- Rehydrate
- Improve circulation
- Improve blood quality

There are several categories to the aging process, some of which you'll recognize from earlier chapters, but consider this a review/overview:

Genetics – Throughout this book I've talked about an individual's genetics. We cannot control our genetics, but we can control how they operate and express themselves. For example, if we have a mutation that increases our risk for autoimmune disease, and this can be turned on by inflammation, then let's keep our inflammation down so the gene will not express.

Toxins — These pesticides/herbicides/infections/ mold/mycotoxins/antibiotics all will affect our cells in a very detrimental way.

Diet — Eating a diet that allows the inflammation nightmare to affect us. Sugar is a highly inflammatory molecule that increases inflammation, causing disturbance to our cells. It creates free radicals, small molecules that cause damage both intracellular and extracellular.

Hormonal Changes — Hormonal changes affect how we age. Personally, I don't think we should keep our hormones as they were when we were eighteen, but we can slow the process of their progressive decline.

Telomeres Length Shortening — This process happens with cell replication, and we now have supplements that will help prevent the shortening of our telomeres, thus preventing rapid aging.

(Telomeres are the end caps to the terminals. Telomerase is a ribonucleoprotein that adds the nucleotide TTAGGG to the 3` end of telomeres. When these telomeres shorten, aging is accelerated.)

Immune System — Oftentimes we eat things that will inhibit our immune system. I hate to keep badgering about sugar, but sugar suppresses our immune system and also feeds our cancer cells; these cancer cells are bombarding every single individual.

Inflammation – Cellular inflammation will turn on the TNF-1 epigenetic gene. Turning this on will increase one's risk for cancer and inflammatory diseases such as lupus, Crohn's, and many other autoimmune diseases. Chronic inflammation can cause lung problems and heart disease. In my practice I have found some amazing things to decrease inflammation, helping to prevent the diseases associated with increased inflammation.

If you remember from my story, I had severe problems and was diagnosed with Crohn's at the age of seventeen.

At this young age they wanted to surgically remove a large portion of my bowel. I took matters into my own hands and began to change my diet. I didn't know it then, but the diet I changed to took out a lot of the inflammatory foods. These foods were causing more and more problems. I later found out other products that helped to remove my inflammation.

I don't believe in an instant cure or some magic potion, but there are other ways to turn back the clock. One is through supplementing with antioxidants, agents that in fact need glutathione in our bodies to perform their actions. Glutathione, as already stated, is the strongest antioxidant known to man. Other antioxidants include grape seed, resveratrol, carotenoids, vitamin E, vitamin C, alpha lipoic acid, CoQ10, and xanthophylls.

All of these are important, and the best way to get antioxidants is through your diet. However, this is not always possible and we should probably use supplements when we are not getting enough antioxidants.

What Role Do Antioxidants Play?

Antioxidants decrease our oxidative stress. Oxidative stress accelerates our aging process and can cause the disease process to start.

Antioxidants are a class of molecules capable of inhibiting the oxidation of another molecule. Our bodies will naturally circulate nutrients due to anti-oxidant properties. The body will also manufacture antioxidant enzymes to control free radical chain reactions. Some antioxidants are produced in our bodies, but others must be injected. To introduce the ones naturally produced in our bodies we must make sure we are injecting the precursors for the specific antioxidant. These antioxidants will help to prevent damage from free radicals.

For true anti-aging, cell health must be taken into account. I truly believe anti-aging starts from cellular health. To do this we optimize the body according to our genetics—how our genetics affect each cell and how each cell affects the organ, the organ system, then the triad, and finally the body as a whole.

A Healing Path to Optimization

Let me restate this because I believe it is important; I don't care if you have arthritis, Alzheimer's, depression, cardiovascular disease, fatigue from whatever cause, gastrointestinal problems, infections, Lyme, MS, parasites, Parkinson's, restless leg syndrome, or you just want to slow down your aging process for optimal health and preventions. *First we take into account your genetics.* Do you have a genetic mutation putting you at risk for Alzheimer's, diabetes, cancer, Parkinson's, MS, or other things? Do you have a genetic mutation not conducive to specific supplements?

After we take into account your genetics, optimize your diet, add the right supplements, and remove toxins to keep your genetic mutations from causing expression (eliminating inflammation that permits these genetics to create havoc in our bodies), secondly, we take into account every cell.

Toxins, as we have seen, will affect all cell components, especially the cell membrane and mitochondria. What if you have genetic mutations that can affect your mitochondria? Well, these areas need proper nutrition, proper fats, vitamins, minerals, and amino acids to bring health healing and preventing diseases that are possible for you.

Thirdly, all these cells make up an organ. The organ's function is taken into account for that organ to be healthy and work optimally. This can be a brain, heart, kidney, bowel, or even adrenals. Each of these has a triad of effects such as the bowel affecting the brain and much more. Knowing how these organs interact and affect one another is how we optimize the organ system.

Lastly, we optimize you as a person, as the organ system affects the entire being. So for prevention and optimization we must take into account all aspects of the person from mental health, hormones, disease process, cellular health, organs, and organ systems. I believe it takes understanding the cell and the entire mechanics of the body to be healthy and bring health to the individual.

If you want true health, start by finding a doctor who understands both traditional and integrative medicine, someone who has spent time studying integrative medicine. Too many doctors hide behind the shingle "Integrative Medicine" but in fact know little about it. If your doctor is not reading articles every week to gain knowledge, then he or she is not the person for you. I personally read five to ten articles per week, sometimes more, because my patients also want me educated; I will even read the articles they present to me.

Let us all humble ourselves and realize we do not and cannot know it all, but we can continue to learn and gain knowledge. It is best for my patients and for me to continue to learn because some things become quickly outdated by new studies and research. I believe we should all collaborate together for the best of all individuals.

My friends, get your life back, one cell at a time, and remember to live—but don't just live, live excellently.

Chapter 12

A Note to Patients and Caregivers: The Healing Journey Begins with You

—⚬⚬⚬—

As this book draws to a close, I want to talk directly to both patients and caregivers because chronic illness never affects only one person—it affects those around the chronically ill person, and most of all the primary caregiver. That caregiver is often not a paid professional but a mother or father, son or daughter, husband or wife; it may even be a close friend.

Regardless of how you came to be ill, your life undoubtedly took a tailspin and normal life may be a distant memory at this point. Perhaps you've been sick for so long you don't even remember what it feels like to be healthy and whole. But I'm here to tell you that whole body health is your God-given birthright. For many of you, that birthright has been stolen. It's time to take back what is yours and finish your days in vibrant, meaningful living.

In the sections below, I've invited my wife, Michelle, to offer insights to both patients and caregivers. Prior to our marriage, she was married to a man diagnosed with incurable brain cancer, and she found herself forced into the role of caregiver in the prime of her life. The wisdom and experience gleaned in those heartbreaking years stand her in good stead today as she works alongside me at Excellent Living. She gets what it's like to be a caregiver, and her naturally compassionate nature is immediately apparent to our patient-clients as well.

Patients

Dr. Crozier: If you've been struggling with illness for a long time, you can find yourself frustrated and very angry with life—feeling agitated, hopeless, wondering if life is worth living. I remember when I was having horrendous burning pain in my feet and legs, and I would lash out in anger at Michelle. But it was so wrong. She was the one giving me security and helping to direct me in the paths I needed to go. So I urge patients to be very cognizant of this. Sickness does not give us a position to lash out. There's a reason behind the anger, certainly, but our actions are a choice.

Michelle: I used to tell Donald, "It's okay to be mad. It's just not okay to stay there." We've encountered so many people who have seen so many doctors and have been sick for so long they've got a wall up. I can spot them. They feel entitled to the sickness, so basically they have surrendered who they are to the identity of the sickness. They excused who they are and have *become* the sickness. They treat the staff that way and they treat Dr. Crozier that way. Being thankful and hopeful is going to get the best results for any treatment.

Dr. Crozier: Remember that emotions are a powerful force. They are going to change the pathways in your body upward toward a healing mode or downward toward a sick mode. Your emotions will also affect your physician's ability to bring healing to your body. You can't have a thought process without having a reaction. When you react on those thoughts, those thoughts become habits and cause a reaction in your life.

I used to struggle with this myself, but I became a survivor because I had to overcome that negativity in thinking I was entitled to receive compassion from people and that the world should treat me differently. I'm still in the changing process—this is not something that goes away quickly if you're a negative person or consumed with being sick.

Michelle: Sick people expect to receive healing in the midst of their negativity. They don't realize they're trying to put two worlds together—health and healing, and destructive negativity. The two are total opposites.

Dr. Crozier: After twenty-five years of practicing medicine, it's my opinion that those who get better and have a healing process in hand are those with a mindset focused on thankfulness, positive things, and hope. Above all else, they have a belief in hope. I've seen many patients who have not received their optimized health because of fear, anger, unbelief, blaming—all the negative things. Some will actually fear being well because they don't know what to do with their lives. The illness has become a crutch, even their whole identity. *What will I do when I'm well?* they ponder. It takes courage to embrace your healing.

Many times I suggest counseling alongside of treatment because it goes hand-in-hand with a patient's road to recovery. Apart from counseling, there are things you can do to promote your own healing process.

Jump-Start Your Own Healing
Here's what I recommend people do on a personal daily basis.

- **Start each day visualizing yourself healthy.** Think about what that looks like. If you're a writer, write down what that looks like. If you can't write, verbalize it. Look at yourself in the mirror and say, "I am healthy, I am well, I know I have a purpose in life."

- **Paste positive affirmations or scriptures** wherever you will see them all day long: bathroom mirror, refrigerator, car dashboard, etc.

- **Only focus on the good that's happening in your life**. You may think nothing is good right now, but if you can wake up and breathe, be thankful for that. Just be thankful for even the small things. So many people are too busy thinking about their sickness. When you focus on the sickness, the sickness and the things that are bad have control of you—your negativity empowers that. And because cells have vibration, you are empowering the bad cells to become more powerful. If you speak *life* and *healing* to your body, mind, and soul, you empower the good cells to become stronger. There's a saying that goes, "Whatever you feed gets stronger." Feed the good things in your life.

- **Choose healthy foods.** This is something you can control rather than giving your sickness control.

- **Take charge of your own care**. If you are able to communicate, be the one to set appointments, discuss your symptoms and changes in your plan of care, take your supplements, etc. As a physician, I desire a relationship with the patient, and this helps me to know exactly which way I need to go with their treatment. But I do understand when care-givers need to be present and give a majority of the history due to the severity of the disease(s).

Finally, seek out integrative physicians who are knowledgeable in the field you need, and seek out somebody who incorporates body, mind, and spirit. If you need help in navigating your healthcare, Excellent Living will be more than happy to refer you toward the best suitable arrangement for you.

Caregivers

Michelle: As hard as it is to be a caregiver, when you get to the place of recognizing that it's a *privilege*, you have embraced your role and released all expectations to the person who is sick—letting them know that you don't expect anything from them.

Caregivers start giving care because they think it's their role: it's what a wife does, or it's what a mother does, and so on. But then it becomes a twenty-four-hour job and it consumes their life. Their life is now all about taking care of the sick one. You can get lost in it all and feel that you no longer matter. Whenever people call the house, they are calling about the sick one; if they visit, it's for the sick one.

When you get to the point of recognizing that it's a privilege—that it's an honor to take care of this person—you're in a place of release. You are at a restful place and a peaceful place.

I always advise caregivers that whenever you're out with the sick one, always have a Plan B. Learn to be flexible, but at the same time learn to say no and not be an enabler. You have to do what is physically, mentally, and spiritually best for that patient.

When the patient is irritable, for example, learn to pull away and make sure you take care of yourself. Have outside activities. Whatever you enjoy doing, do it—whether it's reading or strolling through a garden or taking your pet somewhere. Do whatever helps to restore what keeps pulling at you every day.

**Keep Your Own Identity—
Who You Are Matters Too**
Do not find your identity in caring for the patient. Learn how to release your role. Remind yourself that this is not going to be for the rest of your life. The people who keep their own identity and don't get wrapped up too tight in the caregiving role don't develop codependency. And that's a very good thing.

Always remember to:

• Keep your own identity
• Keep your patience by staying non-reactive
• Take time for yourself away from caregiving

- Tell the patient the positive things that are going on
- Remind the patient, "When you get better, what are your future goals?"

It boils down to this: why would a patient fight for healing if they have everything handed to them and no reason to get any better?

Chapter 13

A Final Word about Genetics

—ᗰ—

We are born with our DNA, something that cannot be changed. Even though we can't change our genetic codes, we *can* work around them. Why does it seem that today we have more genetic mutations than in the past? My theory is completely my own, and I don't know if anyone else agrees with me or not, but let me deposit my beliefs here.

A study commissioned by an environmental group that encompassed five different laboratories obtained umbilical cord blood from babies. The study found two hundred chemicals in each newborn's cord blood. The developing fetus is very vulnerable to environmental toxins. As a person develops these toxins will alter or change the DNA by getting to the very center of every cell. These affected infants, after birth, will now have a greater possibility of developing different diseases throughout their lifetime. The harsh truth: they're starting life at a deficit.

Lessons from Toxic Cats

I have heard Dr. Lee Cowden (one of the integrative physicians treating Lyme) quote a study about feeding cats a bad diet, and those cats eventually became sick. Then the lab began feeding them a good diet and the cats got well. This study continued; they fed the cats a bad diet and the cats became sick again. Those sick cats had offspring who were born sick. After their birth the lab began feeding the kittens a good, healthy diet and they became well. The researchers continued this routine with the third generation of cats, and when the sick cats gave birth and continued a toxic eating pattern, the third generation of cats did not get well when they were fed a good and healthy diet.

We in America are now well into the third and fourth generation of toxic overload and poor diets. There is also a Toronto study revealing many toxins present in utero. These toxins are driven deep into the cells of a developing fetus with rapid cell division.

We know that many individuals with gene mutations that could cause them to the develop cancer, lupus, Crohn's, ulcerative colitis, and many other diseases can be kept healthy by removing the toxins' influencers and holding down inflammation.

The medical website PubMed has an article showing inflammation changing or turning on the pathways for our genes to begin expressing. This in turn will permit our bodies to produce the dreaded disease. By now you are asking: What disease were you genetically born with? Where are you genetically weak? How can you prevent this weakness from expressing?

I have seen in many people's histories that *their disease will progress when toxins and inflammation are left unchecked*. These get caught in areas of the cell that will permit mutations and allow the weak genes to express. This creates a deadly environment. In my work with these individuals, when inflammation is calmed down and toxins are removed, symptoms will often resolve.

Exploring the New Frontier of Genetics-Based Medicine

I could fill volumes with each specific disease and subsets of genetic mutations that some call SNPs, or single nucleotide polymorphisms—a scientific word for a DNA sequence variation. In my research as an integrative physician, I continue to find new genetic information that relates to many individual problems. Every single week I discover research articles not previously published about breakthroughs in the genetic world.

This ongoing research and search for knowledge excites me. You could call it the next frontier in medicine. We've depended on allopathic treatment protocols for *many* years, so clearly it's beyond time for this seismic paradigm shift I referenced in the Introduction.

When I put this all together, I realize our genetics control *a lot*, more than we ever suspected. Genetics control much of our brain activities and how our bodies function. Therefore genetics, I believe, is one of the major factors that needs to be taken into consideration whenever we're treating sick individuals.

To give you an idea of how genes play a role in disease (and disease prevention), estrogen dominance from certain genes (RS1048943, RS762551, RA1056836, RS1000440, RS10012, RS12248560) makes these genes especially prone to expressing symptoms of breast engorgement or maybe even breast cancer. There is also a new theory that prostate cancer is not related to testosterone but to estrogen. It's possible that men who develop prostate cancer have these genetic glitches.

There are specific genes related to dementia such as Hu, Mata, CV2, GAD65, CASPR2 that are primarily due to autoimmune dementia. One of my patients who revealed the symptoms of rapid-progression dementia had those symptoms stopped in their tracks when we took the toxins out and controlled inflammation.

Not surprisingly, genes are even noted in how individuals will metabolize certain drugs, either too fast or too slow.

In my practice I see that a lot of my patients with increased inflammation have defaults in their gluta-thione pathways. As discussed earlier, this is our master antioxidant—and a very important tool to know how to guide through our bodies when we fail to produce enough on our own.

Disease prevention and anti-aging need to be renovated, not just to changing our diet, which is good, but to knowing which genetic factors play a role for us. When we know this we can tailor a diet that's good for our genetics and take specific supplements that benefit our genetics. We don't need to be afraid of our genetics but rather let it empower us. We can be empowered to create an environment that's good for our genetics.

We can alter our supplements, which will in turn enhance our individual makeup and permit us to heal and enhance every cell and organ of our bodies. I am excited about changing pathways, changing genetic expression, changing the cell's ability to heal.

My hope and prayer is that we all will take this endeavor so we can optimize, prevent, and heal one cell at a time.

Endnotes

—ɯ—

1 http://www.prb.org/Publications/Articles/2002/
   JustHowManyBabyBoomersAreThere.aspx
2 http://www.history.com/topics/baby-boomers
3 http://www.popsci.com/scitech/article/2008-01/
   do-cells-make-noise
4 There are multiple articles in PubMed on this, including
   "How sound affects us physically, mentally, emotionally,
   and spiritually" by David Gibson, "The Natural Healing"
   by Dudley Evenson, "The Sacred Geometry of Sound and
   Vibration," and "Wholetones: The Sound of Healing," by
   Michael S. Tyrrell.
5 http://www.freeradical.org.au/education.php?page=6
6 http://articles.mercola.com/sites/articles/archive/2013/
   03/07/inflammation-triggers-disease-symptoms.aspx
7 http://www.caltech.edu/news/microbes-help-produce-
   serotonin-gut-46495
8 http://robbwolf.com/2012/04/09/real-deal-adrenal-
   fatigue/
9 Ibid.
10 Ibid.
11 Ibid.

12 http://en.wikipedia.org/wiki/Epigenetics
13 *The Lancet*, 11 October 1997, volume 350 (9084)
14 French cohort study and Denmark studies, both published in PubMed
15 http://jonbarron.org/article/nature-aging-part-1#
16 Ibid.

About the Author

—◊◊◊—

Dr. Gordon Crozier is the Medical Director of Excellent Living in Orlando, Florida, where he also practices medicine. A board certified physician in the state of Florida, Dr. Crozier graduated from Des Moines University & College of Osteopathic Medicine and Surgery in 1994 with a Doctorate of Osteopathy. After serving his internship and residency in Obstetrics and Gynecology at the Michigan State University Garden City Hospital Campus, he practiced in the areas of neurology, neurosurgery, hormone replacement, and women's health.

To inquire with Dr. Crozier and his staff about your health, please visit www.excellentlivingmed-center.com.

To order a God's Imprint genetic test kit, please visit www.GodsImprint.com.

CPSIA information can be obtained
at www.ICGtesting.com
Printed in the USA
LVOW04*2313110416
483126LV00005B/7/P